PHYLLIS SPEIGHT

HOMOEOPATHY:
------------------------------⊙------------------------------
A HOME PRESCRIBER

SAFFRON WALDEN
THE C.W. DANIEL COMPANY LIMITED

Other Books by Phyllis Speight

Arnica The Wonder Herb
Before Calling the Doctor
Comparison of the Chronic Miasms
Homoeopathy – A Practical
Guide to Natural Medicine
Overcoming Rheumatism & Arthritis
Pertinent Questions & Answers
about Homoeopathy
A Study Course in Homoeopathy
Homoeopathic Remedies for Children
Homoeopathy for Emergencies
A Travellers' Guide to Homoeopathy
Homoeopathic Remedies for
Ears, Nose & Throat
Homoeopathic Remedies for Women's Ailments
Tranquillisation: The Non Addictive Way
Coughs & Wheezes

First published in Great Britain in 1992
by The C. W. Daniel Company Limited
1 Church Path, Saffron Walden
Essex, CB10 1JP, England

© Phyllis Speight 1992

ISBN 0 85207 262 7

Designed by Peter Dolton
Production in association with
Book Production Consultants, Cambridge
Typeset by Rowland Phototypesetting, Bury St Edmunds
Printed and bound by St Edmundsbury Press,
Bury St Edmunds, Suffolk

CONTENTS

Introduction

Many years ago *Essentials of Homoeopathic Prescribing* was written by Dr H. Fergie-Woods and was in constant demand but it was allowed to go out of print and recently my husband suggested that I should revise it.

It was written for the novice rather than for trained homoeopaths, giving the essential symptoms of about eighty remedies as brought out in the provings.

After careful thought I had doubts about my revising another author's work and frankly, did not know where to begin!

However, I appreciate what Dr Fergie-Woods has written and gave the suggestion further thought. Finally I decided to get together a new book, omitting remedies that I considered unsuitable for the untrained, and adding several more that are in common use.

Also, I felt that a little more information about each remedy would be helpful.

Obviously this is not a full materia medica but one that I hope will ease the student into the larger and more detailed volumes.

I would stress that I have tried to give the most important symptoms which help to differentiate one remedy from another together with their characteristics and modalities.

Remedies are like people – you can get to know them! It's a fascinating study.

Phyllis Speight
Devon, 1992

How to use this book

The correct remedy can only be found when the correct information has been obtained from the patient.

In order that the novice or student may prescribe for acute conditions that crop up in every household details under the headings of the Three Legged Stool will point the way.

The three legs, LOCATION, SENSATION and MODALITY must comprise well-marked symptoms. If the answers are hesitant or doubtful forget them.

LOCATION

Write down the EXACT part of the body that is causing problems. This must be done as accurately as possible. For instance, it is not sufficient to put 'head' if a headache is to be cured; there are well over one hundred remedies in Kent's *Repertory* (the book that guides us to the remedy in the materia medica) under 'Head, pain in,' and we have to find the most similar! So we put down the part of the head affected, where the actual pain or discomfort is felt. The more specific we can be about the seat of the trouble the better.

SENSATION

The second leg is the sensation felt, the ache or pain or feeling; this should be described IN THE PATIENT'S OWN WORDS. We must never guess because we don't know the feelings of others (even our own children) and we must not try to help by suggesting words to the one who is suffering. The sensation could be burning, pressing, itching, a feeling of fulness, exhaustion or fear, and so on.

MODALITY

The third leg, Modality, qualifies the symptoms so that anything that makes the symptom better or worse is a modality, e.g., weather, cold, heat, eating, drinking, movement, sleep and so on.

There is a fourth factor which can be helpful and useful if known, and that is CAUSE.

The following three cases will, I hope, be helpful illustrations:-

A friend rang complaining of a headache. I ascertained that it was situated in the forehead, more on the right side; she felt a fullness which developed into a throbbing pain, which was worse from any noise or light and lying down, better from pressure. This gave a picture of *Belladonna* and two doses of the 30th potency removed all traces of the discomfort.

A young man complained of feeling sick, and his stomach was worse from any pressure, he felt nauseated and wished he could be sick as he thought that would make him feel better. He was chilly and irritable. Worse from anything cold and better by warmth. These symptoms are all found under *Nux vomica* and a dose or two put him right very quickly.

A young mother telephoned because her little girl had come home from school not wanting any tea (which was unusual): her face was very flushed and she had a temperature. Her eyes were red and she complained that her ear was hot and painful. It was a very cold day with a sharp east wind blowing and the child had been in the playground at lunch time without any covering on her head.

She was soon tucked up in bed and asleep after a dose of *Aconite*. A second dose when she roused later that evening cleared up all the symptoms because *Aconite* is the remedy for symptoms following exposure to cold wind.

If we prescribe for acute cases quickly and effectively we can so often stop more serious conditions from developing.

ABOUT HOMOEOPATHIC REMEDIES
AND POTENCIES

It is important that homoeopathic remedies should be of good quality and prepared by a firm experienced in this special branch of pharmacy and it is advisable to purchase the products of a well-established firm.

Homoeopathic remedies are sensitive and it is essential that they should be stored in a drawer or cupboard away from sunlight and strong smelling perfumes, soaps etc., and they should not be taken directly after cleaning the teeth with a flavoured toothpaste.

They are available in various forms; tablets and pills are the most popular and they should be handled as little as possible. One pill or tablet is sufficient as a dose (more would have no greater effect) and, where possible, it should be shaken into the cap of the bottle and popped under the tongue where it will dissolve. It should not be swallowed nor washed down with liquid.

In acute troubles the remedy may be given frequently in the 6th. or 12th. potency – half hourly or even more often if necessary but usually one or two hourly is adequate; this depends entirely on the severity of the condition. The golden rule is to allow each dose to work and repeat only when improvement has ceased. When a remedy seems to have ceased to function yet is still indicated, a dose of the 30th. potency might clear the case. However, the higher potencies such as the 30th. 200th. etc., are deep-acting and should be used with great caution and where possible should be prescribed only by an experienced practitioner.

If after a reasonable time the remedy does not appear to work go over the symptoms again to make sure that the remedy corresponds. Do not change the prescription too rapidly – it is of the greatest importance to select the most 'like' medicine and where there is no sign of improvement a doctor should be consulted without delay.

REMEDIES AND THEIR ABBREVIATIONS

Aconite   **Acon.**
Alumina   **Alum.**
Apis Mellifica   **Apis.**
Arnica Montana   **Arn.**
Arsenicum Album   **Ars.**
Belladonna   **Bell.**
Borax   **Bor.**
Bryonia   **Bry.**
Calcarea Carbonica   **Calc.**
Caulophyllum   **Caul.**
Causticum   **Caust.**
Chamomilla   **Cham.**
China (Cinchona)   **China.**
Cimicifuga   **Cim.**
Cocculus   **Cocc.**
Conium   **Con.**
Gelsemium   **Gels.**
Graphites   **Graph.**
Ipecacuanha   **Ip.**
Kali Carbonica   **Kali C.**
Kreosote   **Kreos.**
Lachesis   **Lach.**
Lilium Tigrinum   **Lil. T.**
Lycopodium   **Lyc.**
Mercurius Solubilis   **Merc.**
Natrum Muriaticum   **Nat. M.**
Nitric Acid   **Nit. Ac.**
Nux Moschata   **Nux M.**
Nux Vomica   **Nux V.**
Phosphorus   **Phos.**
Platinum   **Plat.**
Podophyllum   **Pod.**
Pulsatilla   **Puls.**
Sabina   **Sab.**
Secale Cornutum   **Sec.**
Sepia   **Sep.**
Silica   **Sil.**
Sulphur   **Sul.**

MATERIA
MEDICA

ACONITUM NAPELLUS

CHARACTERISTICS

Fear, anxiety, physical and mental restlessness.
Fright – Aconite has a calming effect.
The sudden beginning of an acute illness with fever, anxiety, restlessness and fear.
Fearful for the future, of death, there are so many fears.
Can vomit with fear.
There is much tension.
Complaints caused by exposure to dry cold winds and weather.

Kent says "Aconite is like a great storm; it comes, and sweeps over, and passes away."

The face of Aconite expresses FEAR, and Aconite will cure ailments from fright, mental or physical. But as Tyler, says "The fears of Aconite are more or less intangible. The known, the definite, has no terrors for Aconite. It has not the fear of poverty of Bryonia, the fear of thunder of Phosphorus, the fear of approach of Arnica. But Aconite has the fear of death, the fear of darkness, the fear of bed, the fear of ghosts."

The head has sensations of heaviness, heat and bursting.

The eyes feel dry and hot; lids red and swollen. Ear problems develop suddenly after being out in severe weather. Very sensitive to noise.

Pain at root of nose, dry, stopped up sensation. Very sensitive to smell.

Deathly pale face on rising, may become dizzy. Cheeks tingle. Neuralgia of face which feels numb and tingling.

Mouth dry; white coated tongue. Thirst for large quantities of cold water. Throat dry and red.

Vomits with fear, sweating, great heat and urination. Urine painful, hot and scanty. There can be retention when patient screams and becomes very restless.

Menses suppressed from fear.

Breathing difficult; cough hoarse, dry with shortness of breath.

Palpitation with anxiety and tingling in fingers. Pulse full, tense and bounding. Numbness and tingling in hands and feet; hands hot, feet cold.

Fever with waves of cold, or heat and cold, with restlessness and thirst.

Has a tendency to drowsiness during the day, often followed by disturbed sleep at night.

Sudden onset of high fever with burning head but rest of body cold. Usually occurs within a few hours of exposure to cold, dry winds.

Pains which are burning, stinging, cutting or stabbing may be severe, and may be accompanied by numbness, tingling formication and sometimes by flashes of heat.

Haemorrhage is another feature, sudden severe bleeding of bright, red blood from nose, rectum or uterus associated with acute mental turmoil.

Aconite should be thought of when symptoms suddenly follow excessive summer bathing in cold water, surgical operations and associated shock.

Any symptom which develops after exposure to dry, cold winds should be dealt with by giving Aconite at once. Very often it aborts a more serious condition but should the symptoms persist then a different remedy must be considered.

MODALITIES

WORSE *Extremes of temperature, especially cold, dry winds; in a warm room; in direct sunlight; from wine or stimulants; lying on affected side; at night, especially around midnight.*

BETTER *In open air; from sleep; after profuse sweating.*

AGARICUS MUSCARIUS

CHARACTERISTICS

Jerking, twitching, trembling and itching are strong indications.
Sensations as though pierced by needles of ice.
Symptoms appear diagonally, e.g. right arm and left leg.

Patient can be very loquacious.

He shows no fear.

Singing, shouting and muttering in delirium.

Dizzy feelings from sunlight.

Headache in morning extending into root of nose with nose-bleed or thick mucous discharge.

Reading difficult as type seems to move.

Double vision. Twitching of lids and eyeballs.

Redness, burning itching of ears as if frozen.

Nose itching inside and outside; nervous movements of nose; nose-bleeds in old people.

Facial muscles stiff and twitching.

Burning itching of both hands as if frozen; hot, swollen, red.

Trembling of hands.

Gastric disturbances with sharp pains in liver area.

Stitching pains in spleen.

Severe bearing down pains, especially after menopause.

Spasms of coughing at night after falling asleep, with expectoration of little balls of mucus.

Cough ends in a sneeze.

Irregular palpitation.

Pain in back with sensitiveness of spine to touch. Twitching of cervical muscles.

Itching of toes and feet as if frozen. Chilblains.

Skin burning, itching, redness and swelling as from frostbites.

Paroxysms of yawning.

Starts, twitches and often wakes up.

Shivering over body from above downwards.

Sweats when walking or on slightest motion.

MODALITIES

WORSE *Open, cold air, after eating, after coitus, in cold weather, before a thunderstorm. Pressure on dorsal spine.*

BETTER *Moving about slowly.*

ALLIUM CEPA

CHARACTERISTICS

Acrid nasal discharge but eye secretion bland.

Neuralgic pains like a fine thread following amputation or injury to nerves.

Think of the effects of peeling an onion and some symptoms of this remedy can be felt!

Headaches from catarrh are mostly frontal and worse in a warm room.

Much burning in eyes with smarting lachrymation. But profuse bland lachrymation often accompanies a cold.

Eyes sensitive to light.

Coryza with frequent sneezing and profuse acrid discharge corroding upper lip.

There is hoarseness with hacking cough made worse by breathing in cold air. Larynx tickles.

Sensation as if larynx is torn.

Oppressed breathing from pressure in mid chest.

MODALITIES

WORSE *Evenings; in warm room.*
BETTER *In open air; in cool room.*

ALUMINA

CHARACTERISTICS

Hasty, hurried, time passes too slowly.
Variable mood, better as day advances.
Impulses when he sees sharp instruments or blood.

Eyes inflamed; burning, dryness, smarting.
> Redness of nose.
> Point of nose cracked; scabs with thick, yellow mucus.
> Throat dry and sore.
> Can swallow only small morsels at a time.
> Potatoes disagree. Craves indigestible things.
> Abdominal complaints are left sided.
> Inactivity of rectum. No desire for stool; even soft stools are passed
with great difficulty. There is painful urging quite a time before stool,
then straining at stool.
> Stools hard, knotty, like sheep's dung.
> Menses scanty, pale, and followed by great exhaustion.
> Leucorrhoea is acrid, profuse and ropy.
> Cough on talking or singing in the morning.
> Dry, hacking cough, with vomiting and difficult breathing; with
frequent sneezing.
> When sitting with legs crossed they feel "asleep."
> Heels feel numb.
> Nails brittle.
> Intolerable itching of skin when getting warm in bed.

MODALITIES

WORSE *Periodically; in morning on waking; afternoon; warm room;*
from potatoes.
BETTER *In open air; damp weather; in evening and on alternate days;*
from cold washing.

AMBRA GRISEA

CHARACTERISTICS

Extreme nervous hypersensitiveness.
Patients weakened by age or overwork.
Music aggravates symptoms.

This remedy is particularly adapted to nervous people of old age and patients who are nervously "worn out."

Extreme nervous hypersensitiveness.

Senile dizziness.

Weeps when hears music.

Tearing pains in upper half of brain.

Hearing impaired.

Hollow, nervous, spasmodic, barking cough coming from deep chest.

Palpitation in chest as from an obstruction.

Distention of stomach and abdomen.

Discharge of blood between periods from any exertion or straining at stool.

Very nervous women who cannot pass a stool or urinate when anyone else is in the room.

Urine turbid.

Itching of scrotum with soreness and swelling.

Feeling in urethra as if a few drops had been passed.

Cramps in hands.

Numbness – usually of fingers.

Cannot sleep from worry, must get up.

MODALITIES

WORSE *Music; presence of strangers; from anything unusual; morning; warm room.*
BETTER *Slow motion in open air; lying on painful part; cold drinks.*

AMMONIUM CARBONICUM

CHARACTERISTICS

A feeling of heaviness in all organs.

This remedy is useful for weak, anaemic, flabby women. Guernsey says "This remedy seems particularly useful in constitutionally delicate women who faint easily. They are weak with deficient reaction and want stimulants like ammonia, musk, alcohol etc."

Stoppage of nose at night with long continued coryza. Cannot breathe through nose.

Think of Ammonium Carb. for a dry coryza, acute or chronic.

Snuffles of children.

There can be nose bleeds when washing the face and after eating.

Diphtheria when nose is stopped up.

Pressing teeth together sends shock through head, eyes and ears.

Much oppression in breathing, worse in warm room.

Weak heart.

Menses too frequent and profuse.

Sleepiness during the day.

Pain in wrist joint where sprained long ago (Tyler).

MODALITIES

WORSE *Evenings; at night and has to breathe through mouth; from cold, wet, weather; wet applications; washing; during menses; from 3–4 a.m.*
BETTER *Lying on painful side and on stomach; in dry weather.*

AMMONIUM MURIATICUM

CHARACTERISTICS

Sensation of coldness in back between shoulders.
Secretions profuse and glairy.
Desire to cry.

Free acrid, watery discharge, corroding lip.

Nose obstructed; stuffy feeling; loss of smell.

Swelling of throat with viscid phlegm.

Hoarseness and burning in larynx.

The coldness between shoulders is not better by covering and is followed by itching. It is usually there when there is a chest infection, with or without a cough.

This remedy should be thought of for constipation when stool is hard, dry, crumbling and very difficult to expel. It is sometimes covered with mucus.

Menses flow more at night.

Shooting and tearing pains in tips of fingers and toes.

There is pain with a sensation as if muscles are contracted or too short.

In sciatica Ammonium mur., is helpful when again there is this sensation of contraction in the tendons and patient is worse while sitting, a little better when walking and entirely relieved when lying down.

Pains in heels as if ulcerated.

Chilliness in evenings after lying down.

MODALITIES

WORSE *Open air.*

BETTER *Head and chest symptoms in morning; abdominal symptoms in afternoon.*

ANACARDIUM

CHARACTERISTICS

Loss and great weakness of memory.

Irresistible desire to curse and swear.

Feels as if he had two wills, one commanding, the other forbidding, to do things.

Suspects everyone and everything around him.

Pain and sensation of a plug in different parts of the body, or constriction around limbs or waist.

Pains in stomach when empty.

There is a moral conflict here with an irresistible desire to curse and sweat and do violent acts countered by a conscious compunction to do right.

Seems in a dream.

Feels there is no reality in anything; as if mind and body are separate.

Has strange ideas that he is two people.

He laughs when things are serious and sometimes remains solemn when something funny happens or is sad.

There is a great loss of confidence, especially before an examination or an ordeal.

Irresolute, cannot make decisions.

Great depression. Suspicious. Brain-fag.

Has an affinity with the alimentary canal; disturbance of gastric secretion; empty feeling in stomach.

Excellent for dyspepsia when pain in stomach comes on only when stomach is empty and relieved by eating. Nash says "It ought often to be given for dyspepsia, for which Nux vomica is so indiscriminately used," when the pain is in stomach only when stomach is empty.

Pain as if plug in intestines.

There is desire for stool but with insufficient action to carry it out. Has a sense of plug in anus causing stoppage.

Itching of anus.

Moisture in rectum.

Intense itching of skin.

Symptoms begin on right side and spread to left.

MODALITIES

WORSE *Cold and cold draughts; exertion; when stomach is empty; from mental effort; hot applications; in the morning.*

BETTER *At rest; evening; while eating.*

Relief from taking food is very marked.

ANTIMONIUM CRUDUM

CHARACTERISTICS

Thickly coated white, very white, tongue.

Derangements from overloading the stomach, especially with fat foods, nausea.

Finger nails grow in splits with horny spots.

Corns and callosities on soles of feet.

Child cannot bear to be looked at.

Fitful, cross.

Feverish conditions at night.

Cannot bear heat of sun.

Exhausted in warm weather.

There is excessive irritability; whatever is done fails to give satisfaction.

Headache after bathing and from disordered stomach.

Canthi (angles of eyelids) raw and fissured. Inflammation of eyelids.

Nostrils chapped and covered with crusts; sore, cracked and scurfy.

Yellow crusted eruption on cheeks.

Cracks in corners of mouth. Tongue coated thick-white as if white-washed. Cancer sores.

Loss of appetite; desire for acid food, pickles.

Kent says that all symptoms seem to centre about the stomach. No matter what the complaint the stomach takes part in it.

"Upsets from overloading the stomach especially with fat food; nausea." – Nash.

Constant belching. Bloated feeling after eating.

Diarrhoea alternates with constipation. Hard lumps mixed with watery discharge.

Cough worse coming into warm room with burning sensation in chest; itching of chest; voice harsh and badly pitched.

Pains in fingers.

Continued drowsiness in old people.

MODALITIES

WORSE *Evening; from heat; heat of sun and radiated heat; acids; wine; water and washing; wet poultices.*

BETTER *Open air; during rest; moist warmth.*

ANTIMONIUM TARTARICUM

CHARACTERISTICS

Great weakness, lassitude.

Drowsiness, debility and sweat.

Sleepiness or sleeplessness.

Great accumulation of mucus in air passages with much rattling and inability to raise it.

Nausea, vomiting with loss of appetite.

Pallor. Pale sunken face.

Lack of thirst.

Irritability.

Everything is a burden to this patient – doesn't want to be bothered; which causes him to be irritable, anxious and restless.

Children cannot bear to be touched by strangers and cling to parents and friends.

Patient is chilly but cannot stand a hot, stuffy room or wearing too much clothing.

Feels better for cool, fresh air.

Coated, pasty thick white tongue.

Face pale, covered with cold sweat.

Incessant quivering of chin and lower jaw.

Nausea, retching and vomiting. Thirst for cold water, little and often, and desire for apples, fruits and acids generally.

Great rattling of mucus but very little expectorated.

Coughing and gaping consecutively.

Oedema and impending paralysis of lung.

"For children, invaluable in diseases of the chest where the cough is provoked whenever the child gets angry, which is very often." – Farrington.

Marked wheezing when child breathes.

Violent pain in sacro-lumbar region.

Sensation of heavy weight in coccyx dragging downwards.

Pustular eruption.

Great drowsiness.

MODALITIES

WORSE *Evenings; lying down at night; warmth; in damp, cold weather; from all sour things and milk.*

BETTER *Sitting erect; from eructation and expectoration; fresh air.*

APIS MELLIFICA

CHARACTERISTICS

Jealous and suspicious.

Whining; tearfulness.

Awkward, often drops things.

Constricted sensations.

Oedema.

Pains stinging and burning.

Alternately dry and hot or perspiring.

Thirstlessness; sweats without thirst.

Kent says "Apis is full of dropsy, red rash, eruptions, urticaria, erysipelas . . . in all these there is stinging and burning; burning like coals of fire at times and stinging as if needles or small splinters were sticking in."

There is emotional instability and like the bee who flits from flower to flower, this patient flits from one idea to another.

There is a desire for company.

Fear is quite marked, especially of illness, and of straining something when coughing.

Patient is sad, depressed, tearful; can be very irritable; or joyless and indifferent.

There is great sensitivity to the least contact and aversion to any constriction.

Very drowsy; screams and sudden starting from sleep. Brain feels tired.

Swellings may occur almost anywhere, inflamed and red, or

oedematous; pale and waxy looking or with a transparent appearance of the skin. Skin sore and sensitive.

Apis is a great throat remedy with the Apis swelling, oedema, aggravation from heat plus burning and stinging pains.

There may be a feeling in any part of the body that it is swollen or bruised, or of internal trembling.

Complaints mostly start with violence and rapidity; often on the right side and spread to the left. Pains tend to wander.

Puffy bags (of water) sometimes appear under eyes. Lachrymation is hot.

Suffocative feeling as if he could not draw another breath.

Abdomen extremely tender.

Anus seems open.

Pains occur in legs and arms with pricking and burning sensations. Hands and feet feel swollen, numb, and tremble. Toes are red and burning although feet feel cold.

Sequelae of eruptive diseases when eruptions fail to develop.

MODALITIES

WORSE *From heat in any form (weather, hot rooms, hot bath); from getting wet; touch; pressure; lying down; at about 5 p.m.; during the night, after sleep.*

BETTER *Cool air; open air; cold applications; changing position; sitting up; walking about.*

Argentum Nitricum

CHARACTERISTICS

Fear, anxiety, apprehension regarding future events.

Funks examinations.

Fears failure. Tummy turns over.

Irrational thoughts and imaginations.

Impulsive, does things in a hurry; walks fast.

Claustrophobia.

Looking from heights causes giddiness, looking up at high buildings also causes trouble.

When in a theatre or other gathering seeks a seat which will enable him to make a quick exit or escape.

Dreads crowds.

Irresistible desire for sugar and sweet things which aggravate and cause diarrhoea.

"This patient is irrational, does strange things, and comes to strange conclusions; does foolish things. Disturbance in memory – disturbance in reason." – Kent.

There is great apprehension and fear which promotes hurriedness and restlessness – he is often impelled to walk very fast.

Claustrophobia often ends in panic.

Nervous insomnia; sleep is disturbed by horrible dreams.

Sudden profuse nervous sweats.

Emotional distress or mental exertion brings on physical symptoms.

Feeling of constriction – iron band sensation round chest and waist.

Pains are sharp, and splinter like, which come and go slowly.

Headache with coldness and trembling; a sense of expansion. Aching in frontal eminence with enlarged feeling in corresponding eye. Boring pain, better light bandage or pressure.

Thick mucus – splinter sensation when swallowing.

Strangulated feeling.

Belching accompanies most gastric ailments.

Painful swelling in pit of stomach. "Full of ulceration, especially on internal parts and mucous membranes." – Kent.

Craves sweets.

Ulceration of stomach with radiating pain.

Colic in abdomen with much flatulent distention.

Stool green like chopped spinach.

Fluids go right through him.

Rigidity of calves.

MODALITIES
WORSE *Warmth in any form; at night; from cold food; sweets; after eating; at menstrual period; from emotions; left side.*
BETTER *Fresh air; cold; pressure; eructations.*

Arnica Montana

CHARACTERISTICS
In serious illness says there is nothing the matter with him/her.
After traumatic injuries.
Sore, lame bruised feeling.

Head and face hot, body and extremities cold.
    Bruising.
    Taste, eructations and stool like rotten eggs.

Recent and remote affections from injuries.

Haemorrhage – the result of mechanical injuries.

The results of bruising of the soft parts.

Weakness and weariness as of being bruised.

Everything on which he lies feels hard because of bruised sensation.

Arnica removes shock and trauma following physical injuries.

Many small boils, one after another, which are very painful and very sore.

Prevents suppuration and promotes absorption.

Soreness of parts after labour; prevents haemorrhages.

Peculiar symptoms – mental and physical – Tyler.

Cold nose.

Head burning hot with cold body.

Forgetfulness; absent mindedness.

Sudden horror of instant death.

Fear of being touched.

MODALITIES

WORSE *Least touch; motion; damp cold; wine.*

BETTER *Lying down or with head low.*

ARSENICUM ALBUM

CHARACTERISTICS

Great anguish and restlessness.

Fear, fright and worry.

Prostration yet marked restlessness from anxiety making patient change places constantly.

Great exhaustion after slightest exertion.

Fastidious, hates disorder.

Burning pains better by heat but patient always wants head kept cool.

Burning discharges.

Great thirst for small quantities at frequent intervals.

Kent says "Arsenic affects every part of man; it seems to exaggerate or depress all his faculties, to excite or disturb all his functions . . . it has certain prevailing and striking features. Anxiety, restlessness, prostration, burning and cadaveric odours are prominent characteristics. The surface of the body is pale, cold, clammy and sweating."

Periodic burning pains in the head with restlessness.

Scalp itches intolerably.

Eyes burn with acrid lachrymation. Intense photophobia.

There is thin, excoriating, offensive discharge from the ears.

Nose feels stopped up; no better for sneezing; or there may be a thin watery excoriating discharge.

Tearing, needle like pains in face.

There may be gulping up of burning water.

Patient cannot bear sight or smell of food.

Great thirst but drinks little and often.

Ill effects of vegetables, melons and watery fruits.

Liver and spleen enlarged and painful.

Small, offensive dark stools with much prostration, worse at night and after eating and drinking.

Darting pains through upper third of right lung.

Cough dry, especially after drinking.

Expectoration scanty and frothy.

Pulse more rapid in morning.

Skin dry, rough, scaly; worse cold.

Fever intermittent, paroxysms incomplete with marked exhaustion.

Hay fever.

"Arsenicum brings back old suppressed skin troubles to cure them. Even asthma is seen to be cured with the return of an old eruption." – Nash.

MODALITIES

WORSE *Cold air; wet weather; cold drinks; cold applications; night; after midnight, 1 a.m. to 3 a.m.*

BETTER *Warmth (except head); loves and craves heat.*

Aurum Metallicum

CHARACTERISTICS

Wants to commit suicide, thinks he is no good in the world.

Deep gloom and despair.

Over sensitiveness.

A great remedy for bone pains.

Disgust of life – talks of committing suicide.

Dejected, full of grief; imagines he has lost the affection of friends.

Thinks he is not fit for this world.

Peevish, least contradiction makes him angry.

Oversensitiveness, especially to noise.

Violent pain in head, especially at night.

Extreme intolerance of light. Double vision – upper half of objects invisible.

Obstinate foetid discharge from ear.

Nose ulcerated, painful. Putrid smell from obstructed foetid discharges.

Sensation as if heart stopped beating for 2/3 seconds.

High blood pressure. Pulse rapid; feeble; irregular.

Angina pectoris.

Tightness of chest; feeling of weight on chest.

Liver troubles.

Women suffering from prolapse or enlargement of womb.

Pain and swelling of testicles.

Atrophy of testicles in boys.

Nodes and bone pains.

Rheumatism.

MODALITIES

WORSE *In cold weather when getting cold (many complaints come on only in winter); from sunset to sunrise.*

BAPTISIA

CHARACTERISTICS

Confusion of mind.

Suddenness – of attack; of recovery.

Great muscular soreness.

Septic conditions.

The mind is very confused; thinks he is broken or double; tosses about bed trying to put the pieces together.

Head feels too large; heavy and numb.

Face dark, red and besotted; hot, flushed, dusky.

Breath foetid.

Tongue feels burning; ulcerated; streaked down the middle.

Can swallow only liquids. Tonsils and soft palate swollen but there is no pain.

Sinking feeling in stomach. Abdominal muscles sore on pressure with acute pain at intervals.

Bowels rumble; stools very offensive; thin, dark, bloody.

Sense of suffocation when breathing.

Extremities feel sore and bruised; great soreness all over.

Parts rested on feel sore and bruised.

Septic conditions of blood, e.g. malarial poisoning with extreme prostration; fevers.

Tyler says this remedy is for acute conditions and she has found it almost a specific in gastric flu.

MODALITIES

WORSE *Humid heat; fog; being indoors.*

BARYTA CARBONICA

CHARACTERISTICS

Memory deficient; forgets in the middle of a speech. Great mental and bodily weakness.
Childishness in old people.
Sadness – dejection of spirits.
Timid; bashful; cowardly.
Dread of strangers.
Irresolute, constantly changing his mind.
Chilly people, need much clothing.
All symptoms are worse after eating.

This remedy is indicated very often in infancy and in old age – the two extremes; in the dwarfish growth of young children and in the degenerative changes in old people.

Senile dementia; loss of memory; mental weakness. Bashful, averse to meeting strangers.

Mind and body weak.

Feeble and tottering in old age; childishness and thoughtless behaviour.

Head may be disproportionally large for body.

Hardness of hearing; cracking noises; glands around ears painful and swollen.

Takes cold easily; sneezing and swelling of upper lip and nose.

Smarting pains in throat; swollen and suppurating tonsils with every cold which develops after least exposure to cold.

Can only swallow liquids; stinging pains in throat. Swollen glands, nape of neck.

Stomach and abdomen hard and tense, distended.

Tonsillitis acute or chronic often follows suppressed footsweat.

Both young and old suffer from damp, changes in weather and both are sensitive to cold about the head.

MODALITIES

WORSE *While thinking of symptoms; from washing; lying on painful side.*

BETTER *Walking in open air.*

BELLADONNA

CHARACTERISTICS

This remedy stands for HEAT, REDNESS, THROBBING and Burning. Attacks are violent and onset sudden.

Many acute local inflammations; fevers with hot, burning, dry skin so hot that heat can be felt by the hand before it touches the skin.

Very red, flushed face; dilated pupils of the eyes.

Sudden rise in temperature.

Restless sleep from excited mental states which can go on to delirium.

There is often an acuteness of all senses.

Can get very angry.

Tyler says "Violence runs through Belladonna, and suddenness; it is a remedy of sudden acute conditions associated with turmoil in the brain."

A great children's remedy. There is no thirst but lots of anxiety and fear.

Patient is acutely alive and crazed by a flood of subjective visual impressions and fantastic illusions.

Desire to escape. Fury. Acuteness of all senses.

Pain in head with feelings of fullness, especially in forehead; made worse by light, noise, jar, lying down and in the afternoon.

Face bluish-red.

Eyes – pupils dilated; feel swollen; staring; brilliant, dry; burning.

Ears – inflammation of the middle ear; pain causes delirium; child cries out in sleep. Swelling of neck glands; swollen, tender, red.

Nose – bleeding.

Grinding of teeth.

Throat red, burns like fire, worse right side. Tonsils enlarged; throat feels constricted; difficult swallowing. Spasms in throat.

Stomach – great thirst for cold water; dreads drinking.

Urine frequent and profuse.

Female; Sensitive forcing downwards as if all the organs would protrude at genitals. Menses increased, bright red; too early; too profuse. Haemorrhage hot. Menses and lochia very offensive and hot. Mastitis.

Respiration; tickling, short dry cough worse at night.

Hoarse. Larynx very painful. High piping voice. Moaning at every breath.

Skin; dry, hot, burning; heat can be felt before hand touches the skin; redness and paleness of skin.

Fever: Burning, pungent, steaming heat. No thirst with fever.

Sleep: Starting when closing eyes or during sleep.

MODALITIES

WORSE *After 3 p.m. or after midnight; from uncovering, or draught of air and lying down; touch; jar; noise; draught.*

BETTER *Being semi-erect (with head high) and being covered.*

BERBERIS

CHARACTERISTICS

Rapid change of symptoms; pains alter in character and move from one part of the body to another.

Head – Sensation of tight cap pressing upon whole of scalp.

Stomach – Nausea before breakfast.

Stool – Fistula in ano.

Urinary – Urine with thick mucus and bright red, mealy sediment. Pain in thighs and loins on urinating.

Extremities – Neuralgia under finger-nails with swelling of finger joints.

Skin – Itching, burning, smarting; worse scratching. Eczema of anus and hands. Circumscribed pigmentation.

MODALITIES

WORSE *Motion; standing, which brings on, or increases, urinary complaints.*

BORAX

CHARACTERISTICS

Dread of downward motion in nearly all complaints, which brings anxiety.
Very nervous and frightened.
Sensitive to sudden noise.

Tyler says "Borax is another of those invaluable minor remedies with very distinctive symptoms and selective tissue action."

Guernsey says "Great fear of downward motion of every kind. Afraid to go downstairs; can't swing; ride horseback or use a rocking chair. Children spring up suddenly on being laid down in bed; or maybe sleeping quietly when they suddenly wake up screaming and holding on to the sides of the cot, without any apparent cause."

And now, of course, there is often great fear when descending in an aeroplane.

Nervous, anxious, fidgetiness and sensitiveness are prominent symptoms in Borax.

Eye-lashes become gummy and stick together.

Ulcerated sore mouth; mouth is hot.

Cough with expectoration which is offensive.

Soft, light yellow mucus in stool.

White, albuminous, starchy leucorrhoea.

Menses too soon, profuse.

Worse before urination.

Frequently screams before passing urine.

MODALITIES

WORSE *Warm weather.*
BETTER *Cold weather.*

BRYONIA

CHARACTERISTICS

Complaints develop slowly.
Great irritability.
Excessive thirst for copious draughts at long intervals.
Stitching and tearing pains which are worse any movement and better for rest, and from pressure.
Dryness of mucous membranes from lips to rectum.
Faintness when head is raised (sitting up in bed).

Tyler says "Bryonia is one of the priceless remedies of homoeopathy especially useful in acute cases. Bryonia is also a remedy of very definite symptoms that can hardly be missed, therefore it is one of the easiest to prescribe with assurance."

Guernesy says of Bryonia "The great characteristic of this remedy is aggravation produced by any motion."

The Bryonia illnesses come on and progress very gradually rather than abruptly; they follow exposure to cold east winds or change of weather from cold to warm. Anger, a bad fright or resentment may be responsible and it is often a day or two later that symptoms begin to appear.

This type of patient is very fearful about the future although he is always making plans; he is very afraid of poverty. He can get very anxious, irritable and depressed.

When ill he cannot make any effort, even to speak; he wants to be perfectly still and left undisturbed. There is sometimes a wish "to go home" when he is lying in his own bed.

Although symptoms are often caused by exposure to dry cold and cold winds, the patient prefers a cool room, he is unhappy if it gets too warm or if he is too well wrapped up.

There is frequent bleeding of nose when menses should appear.

Lips are parched, dry and cracked.

Dryness of mouth, tongue and throat with excessive thirst for long drinks at long intervals. There is also great dryness of air passages; cough; alimentary canal and stool (when constipated). Cough dry at night, must sit up; worse after eating or drinking, with stitches in chest. Warm room excites cough.

There is pressure in stomach after eating as from a stone; also nausea and faintness when sitting up. Burning stitching pains in abdomen, worse from pressure, coughing and breathing.

Stiffness and stitching pains in back.

Joints red, swollen, hot.

Pains are tearing or stitching, always worse from any movement and soreness of the affected parts which are worse from being touched. But firm pressure brings relief.

Sweating is profuse, sour smelling and worse during the night, especially around 2 a.m.

MODALITIES

WORSE *Heat; hot weather; motion; muscular effort; touch; morning.*
BETTER *Cool air; applications; drinks; lying motionless when very ill; lying on affected side; firm pressure; after sweating.*

CACTUS GRANDIFLORA

CHARACTERISTICS

Sadness; melancholy.
Constrictions as of an iron band, especially around head.
Spasmodic pains.
Periodicity.
Pulseless – panting – prostrated.

Nash says "In any haemorrhages seeming to be in sympathy with heart trouble think of Cactus."

Fears death – believes disease incurable.

Attacks of suffocation with fainting, cold sweat on face and loss of pulse.

Fluttering and palpitation of heart, worse when walking or lying on left side.

Great irregularity of heart action.

Haemorrhage – constrictions – periodicity and spasmodic pains.

Congestive headaches.

Sensations as from a weight on vertex.

Constriction in chest as if bound or from an iron band preventing normal movement.

Endocarditis (inflammation of the lining membrane of the heart) with mitral insufficiency, together with violent and rapid action.

Violent palpitation worse lying on right side and at approach of menses.

Heart troubles sometimes caused by inflammatory rheumatism.

Constriction in stomach.

Persistent sub-normal temperatures.

Oedema of left hand, leg and foot.

Rheumatism of all joints.

MODALITIES

WORSE *At 11 a.m. and 11 p.m.; lying on left side; walking; going upstairs.*
BETTER *Open air.*

CALCAREA CARBONICA

CHARACTERISTICS

Fat; flabby; fair; faint.

A jaded state, mental or physical, due to overwork.

Apprehensive and fearful.

Hand is soft, cool and boneless; gives you the shivers to shake hands with Calacrea.

Everything smells sour; stool, urine, and taste is sour.

Profuse cold, sour sweat, especially on head.

Sweats even in cold room.

Enlargement of glands.

Slow in movement.

Craves eggs and indigestible things like chalk, earth, raw potatoes.

Feels better when constipated.

Feet feel as if wearing cold, damp stockings.

Great sensitivity to cold and cold, damp weather; dreads open air; at the same time cannot bear the sun.

Breathless; walking slowly up a slight hill can bring on sweating and breathlessness.

Tyler says "Some remedies are difficult to spot; the difficulty is to miss Calcarea when typical."

Fear, loss of reason, misfortune. Forgetful.

Icy coldness in and on head, especially right side. Much sweat, wets pillow.

Spots and ulcers on cornea, chronic dilation of pupils.

Muco-purulent inflammation of middle ear and enlarged glands.

Nostrils sore and ulcerated. Polypi. Takes cold at every change in the weather.

Persistent sour taste.

Swelling of tonsils.

Craving for indigestible things – chalk, coal, also eggs, salt, sweets. Frequent sour eructations, sour vomiting. Dislikes fat. Loss of appetite when over-worked. Longs for cold drinks.

Inguinal and mesenteric glands swollen and painful. Distention with hardness. Gall-stone colic.

Sour. Children's diarrhoea.

Frequent emissions.

Menses too early, too profuse, too long, with vertigo; toothache and cold damp feet.

Painless hoarseness. Suffocating spells worse going up stairs or slightest ascent.

Very sensitive to touch, pressure or percussion.

Renal colic.

Cold, damp feet. Soles of feet raw. Tearing in muscles.

Some disagreeable idea always arouses from light slumber.

Chill at 2 p.m. begins internally in stomach region. Night sweats especially on head, neck and chest. Sweat over head in children so that pillow becomes wet.

MODALITIES

WORSE *On waking; morning; after midnight; bathing; working in water; full moon; mental and physical exertion; stooping; pressure of clothes; open air; cold air; cold wet weather; letting limbs hang down.*

BETTER *After breakfast; drawing up limbs; loosening garments; in the dark; lying on back; from rubbing; dry, warm weather.*

CALCAREA PHOSPHORICA

CHARACTERISTICS

Anaemia.

Memory weak; slow to learn.

Abdomen sunken.

Feels complaints more when thinking about them.

Helps anaemic children who are peevish, have cold extremities and feeble digestion.

Nash says "Calc. Phos. has also a very peculiar desire – the little patient instead of wanting eggs wants ham rind – a very queer symptom but a genuine one."

Headache worse near region of sutures; change in weather and of schoolgirls with diarrhoea.

Eyeballs hurt, ache as if beaten.

Nasal polypus.

Slowness in teething.

Chronic enlargement of tonsils.

Adenoids.

Craves bacon, ham, salted or smoked meats.

Much flatulence.

At every attempt to eat, colicky pains in abdomen.

Abdomen sunken, flabby.

Stool – Green, slimy, hot, spluttering with foetid flatus.

Extremities – Stiffness and pains with cold, numb feeling. Rheumatic troubles worse autumn or spring when air is cold and damp. Joints have cold, numb feeling. Excellent for broken bones when they refuse to knit.

Skin – Numbness and crawling sensation.

MODALITIES

WORSE *Cold and every change in weather; by thinking of pain; exertion.*
BETTER *By rest.*

CALENDULA

CHARACTERISTICS

Promotes healthy granulation and rapid healing.
Remarkable healing agent when applied locally.

Lacerated scalp wounds.
Deafness worse damp weather.
Heartburn. Epigastric distention.
In fever, coldness. Great sensitiveness to open air.

MODALITIES

WORSE *In damp, heavy, cloudy, weather.*

CANTHARIS

CHARACTERISTICS

Raw, burning pains.
Intolerable, constant urging to urinate.
Abdominal complaints worse drinking coffee.

Acute mania.
Fiery, sparkling staring look in eyes.
Burning in mouth, pharynx and throat. Great difficulty in swallowing liquids. Very tenacious mucus.
Chest: Tenacious mucus.
Very sensitive, violent burning in stomach, worse drinking coffee.

Stool with shivering and burning. Mucous stools like scrapings of intestines. Bloody with burning and constant straining, with shuddering after stool.

Intolerable urging to urinate.

Urine scalds and is passed drop by drop.

Male: strong desire – painful erections.

Female: Nymphomania (insane sexual desire).

Pleurisy with exudation.

Heart: Pericarditis with effusion.

Eruptions with burning and itching.

Burns scald with rawness and smarting better cold applications, followed by undue inflammation.

Erysipelas.

MODALITIES

WORSE *From touch or approach; urinating; drinking cold water or coffee.*

BETTER *Rubbing.*

CARBO VEGETABILIS

CHARACTERISTICS

People who have never recovered from the effects of some previous illness. Imperfect oxidation.
Sluggish, fat, lazy.

Headache from any over-indulgence.

Hair falls off easily.

Nose-bleeds in daily attacks with pale face.

Stomach: Eructations, heaviness, fullness, sleepiness.

Contractive pain extending to chest with distention of abdomen.

Digestion slow; food putrefies before it digests.

Aversion to fats. Simplest food distresses.

Abdomen greatly distended. Flatulent colic.

Acrid, corrosive moisture from rectum. Bluish burning piles; pain after stool.

Hoarseness worse evenings.

Cough with burning in chest.

Asthma in aged with blue skin.

Limbs go to sleep.

Cold from knees down.

Skin blue, cold, bruised; with moist hot perspiration.

MODALITIES

WORSE *Evening; light and open air; cold; from fat food, butter, coffee, milk, wine; warm damp weather.*
BETTER *Eructations; from being fanned; cold.*

Causticum

CHARACTERISTICS

Intensely sympathetic.
Depression; apprehension; timidity; irritability.
   Aches and pains with soreness, rawness and burning.
   Paralysis of single parts, e.g. face, throat, vocal chords, limbs, from exposure to cold, dry winds.
   Skin dirty white, sallow.
   Tearing pains.
   Burning, soreness and rawness.

Melancholy; sadness; looks on the dark side of everything.
   Vision can be affected; incipient cataracts which Causticum has been known to cure.
   Deafness with noises, roaring, humming etc. Reverberations, especially of own voice.
   Pimples and warts on nose. Coryza with hoarseness.
   Yellowness of face. Stiffness of jaws.
   Tongue coated white on sides, red in middle.
   Gums bleed easily.
   Burning in throat; rawness and tickling with dry cough.
   Retention of urine after surgical operations.
   Uterine inertia during labor.
   "Involuntary passage of urine when coughing; sneezing; blowing nose; at night when asleep; when walking." – Nash.
   Constipation frequent but unsuccessful desire for stool.
   Haemorrhoids swollen, itching, smarting, moist, stinging, burning; raw and sore.
   Menses cease at night, flow only during day.
   Hoarseness with pain in chest. Loss of voice.
   Cough with soreness of chest.
   Cough with pain in hip, especially left, worse evening and warmth of bed; better drinking cold water.
   Contracted tendons; rheumatic tearing in limbs; unsteadiness of muscles in forearms and hands.

MODALITIES

WORSE *In clear, fine weather; dry, cold winds; cold air; from motion of travelling.*

BETTER *Damp, wet weather; warmth; heat of bed.*

CHAMOMILLA

CHARACTERISTICS

Frantic irritability – cannot bear it – whatever it may be!
Impatient; over-sensitive.
Whining restlessness; impatient; snappish.
Is bad tempered when she cannot get what she wants.
Inability to control temper.

This is a great remedy for children, especially when teething – they wake up in pain with often one red and one pale cheek, and warm sweat on head. They toss around, cannot keep still, very restless and irritable, howling with pain which is intolerable.

The same symptoms can, of course, be applied to some adults!

There may be jerking and twitching; everything seems unbearable, pain intolerable.

Everything irritates, nothing pleases.

There can be great melancholy with brooding.

Symptoms which arise from anger, contradiction or interference.

Emotion may cause fainting.

Mental calmness contra-indicates Chamomilla.

One cheek red, hot, the other pale and cold.

Earache, swelling and heat driving patient frantic.

Teeth-ache, worse after warm drink.

Flatulent colic after anger with red cheeks and hot perspiration.

Stool hot, green, watery feotid, slimy with colic.

Profuse discharge of clotted, dark blood with labour-like pains.

Irritable, dry, tickling cough.

Hoarseness, hawking; rawness of larynx.

Pains felt by this patient are quite unbearable and seem out of proportion to any obvious pathological lesion.

MODALITIES

WORSE *From anger; exposure to heat, draughts, winds; before and during menstruation; first part of the night.*

BETTER *Warm, moist, humid weather; riding in a vehicle or (children) being carried.*

CHELIDONIUM

CHARACTERISTICS

Constant pain under inferior angle of right scapula.
Yellow eyes, face, skin, urine.
Tongue thickly coated yellow.

This is a great liver remedy with the very marked symptom of constant pain under inferior angle of right shoulder blade.

It is a right sided remedy.

There may be bilious complications during gestation.

Icy coldness from nape of neck over head which feels extremely heavy.

Neuralgic pains over right eye.

Prefers hot food and drink.

Tongue thickly coated yellow with red margins, showing imprint of teeth.

Nausea and/or vomiting better by drinking very hot water.

Eating temporarily relieves stomach symptoms.

Diarrhoea alternating with constipation.

Icy coldness of tips of fingers.

Skin yellow.

MODALITIES

WORSE *Right side; motion; touch; change of weather; early morning.*
BETTER *From pressure.*

CIMICIFUGA

CHARACTERISTICS

Agitation and pain indicate this remedy.
The greater the flow, the greater the pain.
Great depression with dream of impending evil.

Waving sensation or opening and shutting sensation in brain. Pressing outward pain.

Shooting pains in eyes.

Intense aching of eyeball. Pain from eyes to top of head.

Gnawing pain in stomach.

Menses profuse, dark, coagulated. Pain across pelvis from hip to hip.

Dry, short cough worse speaking and at night.
Stiffness and contraction in neck and back.
Muscular soreness. Intercostal rheumatism.
Rheumatism affecting the belly muscles, especially the larger ones.

MODALITIES

WORSE *Morning; cold; during menses (the more profuse the flow the greater the suffering).*
BETTER *Warmth; eating.*

CINCHONA OFFICINALIS (CHINA)

CHARACTERISTICS

Debility and complaints after excessive loss of fluids; bleeding; periods; diarrhoea.
Haemorrhage can be profuse with fainting.
Periodical affections, especially every other day.

Devoid of poise.
Debility from exhausting discharges.
Mental and emotional symptoms from extreme tiredness and weakness.
Intense throbbing of head.
Pressure in eyes.
Ringing in ears.
Violent dry sneezing.
Flatulence, belching of bitter or regurgitated food gives no relief.
Hiccough.
Distended abdomen.
Undigested, frothy yellow stool but painless.
Dark clots and abdominal distention.
Suffocative catarrh; rattling in chest; violent cough after every meal.
Pains in limbs and joints worse slight touch.
Skin extremely sensitive to touch but hard pressure relieves.
Coldness with much sweat.
Inflammation of skin.

MODALITIES

WORSE *Slightest touch; least draught of air; every other day; after eating.*
BETTER *Hard pressure on painful parts; bending double; open air; warmth.*

Cocculus Indica

CHARACTERISTICS

Extreme irritability of nervous system.
Cannot bear contradiction.
Profound sadness.
Effects of night-watching.
Sensation of hollowness; emptiness.
Time passes too quickly. Slowness in thinking worse after an emotional disturbance.
Sensitive to hot or cold air.

Time passes too quickly.
> Profound sadness.
> Vertigo and nausea when riding in a vehicle or sitting up.
> Headache in occiput (back of head) or nape.
> Aversion to food, drink and tobacco.
> Metallic taste.
> Abdomen distended with wind and feels full of sharp stones when moving. Abdominal muscles weak.
> Purulent gushing leucorrhoea between menses which is very weakening.
> Paralytic pain in small of back.
> Pain in shoulders and arms as if bruised.
> Trembling and pain in limbs.
> Knees crack on motion.
> Chilliness with perspiration and heat of skin.

MODALITIES

WORSE *Eating after loss of sleep (night watching); open air; smoking; riding; swimming; touch; noise; jar; afternoon; menstrual period; after any emotional disturbance.*
BETTER *When lying quiet.*

Coffea

CHARACTERISTICS

Great activity of mind and body with sleeplessness; restless; great sensitivity.
Troubles from sudden surprises.
Very sensitive to pain.

Acts on nervous system.

Unusual activity of mind and body.

All senses more acute; full of ideas.

Lively fancies.

Full of future plans.

Very emotional.

Especially adapted to mental shock, sudden surprise; excessive laughter; disappointed love; to various moods; strong noises; smells; from crying, then laughing then, crying again.

Sleepless on account of mental activity.

Exasperation, tears; tossing about in anguish.

Headache one sided. Seems as if nail were driven into head.

Headache from mental exertion, thinking, talking.

Jerking toothache, better holding ice-water in mouth.

Excessive hunger. Intolerance of tight clothing.

Hyper-sensitive vulva and vagina.

MODALITIES

WORSE *Excessive emotions; strong odours; noise; open air; cold; at night.*

BETTER *Warmth; from lying down.*

COLCHICUM

CHARACTERISTICS

Hypersensitivity.

Smell of cooking nauseates even to the point of fainting.

Great prostration.

Icy coldness in stomach.

This patient is always extremely exhausted when ill; and any pains are intolerable owing to acuteness of all sensations.

The smell of food causes much nausea; there is icy coldness in stomach or, occasionally, violent burning.

Craving for various things which are not wanted when being cooked. Smells bring on nausea.

Much distention of gas in abdomen.

Autumnal dysentery when stool contains white shreddy particles.

Inflammation of big toe and gout in heel which patients cannot bear to have touched.

MODALITIES

WORSE *Exposure to cold and damp, especially to autumn rain; extreme heat; sundown to sunrise; motion; being touched; loss of sleep; mental exertion and smell of cooking.*

BETTER *From warmth; warmly wrapped up and rest.*

COLOCYNTHIS

- -

CHARACTERISTICS

Agonizing pains in abdomen causing patient to bend double.
Sensation as if clamped with iron bands.

Patient extremely irritable; easily angered followed by ill effects. Anger with indignation.

Is better left alone, doesn't want to talk.

Suffers tearing, violent, neuralgic pains (often left sided); in paroxysms, sometimes with faintness and weakness.

Vertigo when turning head to the left.

Sharp, boring pains in eyes better for pressure.

Neuralgia in face with chilliness.

Very bitter taste.

Chilly inside and sensitive to cold; disinclined for food. Constant desire to drink.

Agonizing, cutting pain in abdomen causing jelly-like stools.

Boring pain in ovary; must double-up with great restlessness.

Contraction of muscles.

Cramp-like pain in hip.

Skin hot and dry.

Sweat if present may smell like urine.

MODALITIES

WORSE *From anger and indignation; cold wind; damp cold; eating raw fruit; drinking ice-cold water when hot; suppressed sweat; around 4 p.m.*

BETTER *Bending double; hard pressure; warmth (locally applied heat).*

CUPRUM METALLICUM

- -

CHARACTERISTICS

SPASMS! Spasmodic affections.
Cramps.
Convulsions.
Violent contractive and intermitting pain.
Nausea.

Mental and physical exhaustion from over-exertion of mind or loss of sleep.

Contraction of jaws.

Strong, metallic, slimy taste.

When drinking the fluid descends with gurgling sound.

Abdomen feels contracted.

Spasm and constriction of chest.

In whooping cough children get stiff, breathing ceases, there is spasmodic twitching; after a while consciousness returns, they vomit and recover slowly.

Cramps in calves and soles of feet.

Spasms begin in fingers and toes and spread.

Affections from suppressed skin troubles or loss of sleep.

Skin bluish, marbled.

MODALITIES

WORSE *Before menses; from vomiting; contact.*
BETTER *During perspiration; drinking cold water.*

DROSERA

- -

CHARACTERISTICS

Affects respiratory organs.
Cough with paroxysms following each other rapidly – whooping.

The remedy is first thought of for whooping cough but check to see that symptoms of Drosera fit those of the patient.

Restlessness; changes from one thing to another.

Feels dejected; disheartened and concerned about the future. Anxious; full of mistrust; peevish.

Crawling in larynx which provokes coughing.

Rough, scraping sensation deep down with dryness exciting short cough with yellow, slimy expectoration and hoarseness.

Cough, paroxysms follow each other so quickly patient finds it difficult to breathe.

Cough deep, hoarse, spasmodic until he retches and vomits.

Oppression in chest so that breath cannot be expelled.

Cough worse at night.

Asthma when talking.

Pain in joints.

MODALITIES

WORSE *After midnight; lying down; getting warm in bed; drinking; laughing.*

DULCAMARA

CHARACTERISTICS

Specific relation to skin and glands.

Mucous membranes secrete more profusely while skin is inactive.

Rheumatic problems induced by damp, cold and are worse every change to cold.

Complaints caused by or worse from change of weather from warm to cold.

Mental confusion.

Scaldhead; thick, brown crusts.

Back of head heavy and aches in cold weather.

Nose stuffed up when there is cold rain.

Colds settle in eyes; thick, yellow discharge.

Tearing pain from cheek to ear, eye and jaw, preceded by coldness of parts with great hunger.

Facial neuralgia worse from slightest exposure to cold.

Aversion to food. Great thirst for cold drinks.

Cutting pain around naval.

Stool green, watery, slimy, bloody mucus, especially in summer when it can suddenly become cold; from damp, cold weather.

Must urinate when getting chilled.

Before menses appear a rash develops.

Cough after physical exertion.

Pain in small of back.

Feet icy cold.

Pruritis always worse cold weather.

MODALITIES

WORSE *At night; from cold in general; damp, rainy weather.*
BETTER *From moving about; external warmth.*

FERRUM METALLICUM

CHARACTERISTICS

Oversensitiveness.
Weakness from speaking or walking although looking strong.
Pallor of skin.

Slight noises unbearable. General restlessness.

Congestive headache; hammering and pulsating in head.

Pain in back of head.

Fiery red and flushed face from least pain, emotion, exertion.

Flushed, red face, better slowly walking.

One of very few remedies that has red face during chill.

Pain in teeth, better from ice-cold water.

Voracious appetite.

Regurgitation of food or eructation immediately after eating. Spits up food by the mouthful.

Vomiting immediately after eating and after midnight. Food lies in stomach all day and is vomited at night.

Intolerance of eggs.

Bowels feel sore as if bruised; undigested, painless stools at night or while eating and drinking.

Menses too soon, too profuse, too long lasting with firey red face, ringing in ears.

Flow pale, watery, debilitating.

Pulse full but soft and yielding; also small and weak.

Heart suddenly bleeds into blood vessels.

Chest oppressed.

Cough with vomiting of food.

Chill at 4 a.m.

Local congestions and inflammations.

Profuse haemorrhage from any organ, blood light with dark clots.

Anaemia with paleness of all mucous membranes with sudden fiery, red face.

MODALITIES

WORSE *While sweating; while sitting still; after cold washing and overheating. Aggravation at midnight.*

BETTER *Walking about slowly but weakness obliges patient to lie down; after rising.*

GELSEMIUM

CHARACTERISTICS

Affects more the nerves of motion, causing muscular prostration and varying degrees of motor paralysis.

Dizziness, drowsiness, dullness, trembling.

Tiredness, limbs feel tired; eyelids feel heavy.

Fearful; terrors of anticipation.

Apathy regarding illness.

Dullness; langour; listless.

Apathy regarding illness.

Vertigo spreading from occiput; band feeling around head, and occipital headache. Dull, heavy aching. Pain in temples extending to ears.

Eyelids heavy; dim sighted. Orbital neuralgia with contraction and twitching of muscles.

Face hot; heavy, flushed, besotted looking.

Post diphtheric paralysis of throat. Feeling of a lump, and pain from throat to ear. Spasm of glottis.

Diarrhoea from emotional excitement; cream coloured or tea green.

Profuse, clear, watery urine. Retention.

Painful periods with scanty flow.

Spermatorrhoea (involuntary flow of semen) without erection.

A feeling as if it were necessary to keep in motion or else the heart's action would cease.

Weak, slow pulse of old age.

Excessive weakness and trembling of limbs.

In fever wants to be held, he shakes so.

Aids in bringing out eruptions.

MODALITIES

WORSE *Damp weather; emotion; excitement; bad news; 10 a.m.*

BETTER *Bending forward; open air; continued motion; headache is relieved by profuse urination.*

GLONOINE

CHARACTERISTICS

Local congestions especially to head and chest.
Bursting headache rising from neck, with throbbing and bursting feeling;
worse least jar.
Cannot bear anything on head, e.g. hat.
Sunstroke. Bad effects from being exposed to sun's rays.

"This is one of our great head remedies." – Nash.

Confusion – loss of location in familiar streets, everything looks strange.

Sensation of pulsating through body.

Sensation of blood surging from head to heart.

Head heavy but cannot lay it on pillow.

Throbbing or bursting headache, worse bending head backwards.

Cannot bear any heat about head.

Head must be uncovered; cannot bear a hat.

Throbbing in whole of body.

Violent palpitation of heart with throbbing carotids; pulsating headache in forehead and between temples.

Undulating sensation as if moving in waves.

Farrington says "A tendency to sudden and violent irregularities of the circulation."

Kent says "Sunstroke, sudden congestions to head – cold feels good to head; heat feels good to extremities. When lower limbs are covered with clothing in a cool room and windows open, convulsions are relieved and patient breathes more easily."

MODALITIES

WORSE *Exposure to sun's rays; gas, or open fire; jar; stooping; having hair cut; wine; lying down; from 6 a.m. until noon; left side.*
BETTER *Brandy.*

GRAPHITES

CHARACTERISTICS

Fat, chilly, costive.
Tendency to obesity.
Eruptions oozing thick honey-like liquid.

Nails thick and mis-shapen.
Intolerance of light, especially sunlight.
Always cold but craves fresh air; must be well wrapped up.

Sad, despondent, weeps; thinks of nothing but death.
   Restless, anxious, apprehensive; self pity.
   Unable to make decisions. Flies into a rage but easily consoled.
   Music causes weeping.
   Burning in vertex.
   Eyelids red and swollen; eczema of lids, covered with scales and crusts.
   Dryness of inner ears. Moisture and eruption behind ears. Hearing better in noise.
   Feeling of cobwebs on face.
   Burning in stomach causes hunger. Hot drinks disagree. Constrictive pain. Pain relieved by food or drink; by hot food or drink and by lying down. Tyler says "Graphites has great value in gastric or duodenal ulcer."
   Incarcerated flatulence in abdomen, must loosen clothing.
   Stools offensive; knotty and large. Eczema around anus. Fissure.
   Menses too late. Leucorrhoea pale, thin, profuse, white, excoriating.
   Fingernails thick, black, rough, out of shape.
   Unhealthy skin, every little injury suppurates.
   Eruptions ooze a sticky exudation.
   Tendency to sudden weakness and exhaustion with desire to lie down.
   Numb sensations.
   Left-sided complaints.

MODALITIES
WORSE *Warmth at night.*
BETTER *In the dark; wrapping up.*

HEPAR SULPHURIS

CHARACTERISTICS
Hyper-sensitive to all impressions; to touch, pain, cold air.
Tendency to suppuration.
Coughs when any part of body becomes uncovered.
Feeling as if wind was blowing on some part.
Sweats easily on slight exertion.

"There is no other remedy that I know that has the amelioration so strongly in damp weather as Hepar sulph." – Nash.

Pain intolerable, felt intensely, sometimes causing faintness; sticking, splinter-like.

Very irritable; quarrelsome; difficult to get on with; furious over petty things; never satisfied, wants constant change. Slightest cause irritates.

Sad, depressed or impetuous; impulsive.

Very poor memory.

Eyes – ulcers on cornea.

Hay-fever. Thick offensive discharge from nose smells like old cheese.

Cold sores round mouth very sensitive.

When swallowing sensation of a splinter in throat. Quinsy with impending suppuration.

Cough excited when any part of body is uncovered or gets cold.

Choking cough excited by tightness of breath; dry and deep.

Abscesses of labia with great sensitiveness.

Stool sour, white, undigested, foetid.

Unhealthy skin, every little injury suppurates.

Putrid ulcers surrounded by little pimples. Ulcers very sensitive.

Chronic and recurring urticaria.

Chilly in open air or from slightest draught.

"Sweating all night without relief belong to a great many complaints of Hepar." – Kent.

MODALITIES
WORSE *Cold and cool air; cold dry winds; draughts; cold food or fluids; light touch; pressure; lying on affected side; mornings; evenings, and in winter.*
BETTER *Warmth; warm, wet weather; after a meal.*

HYOSCYAMUS

CHARACTERISTICS
Perfect picture of mania; quarrelsome, obscene character.
Lascivious mania. Desire to uncover.
Nervous agitation
Tremulous weakness and twitching of tendons.
Carries on conversations with imaginary people.

Very suspicious; foolish, inclined to laugh at everything; deep stupor.
Pupils dilated. Constant staring at objects nearby.
Deafness.
Uvula elongated. Inability to swallow.
Foams at mouth.
Tongue dry, cracked, hard or clean, parched white.
Inflammation of stomach. Toxic gastritis.
"Much urging for stool with rare evacuations." – Hahnemann.
Diarrhoea involuntary.
Involuntary urination.
Dry, spasmodic cough at night when lying down which stops as soon as patient sits up only to start again on lying down.
In fevers patient will not remain covered; is violent and active.
Picking at bedclothes.
Great restlessness; every muscle twitches from eyes to toes.

MODALITIES

WORSE *At night; during menses; after eating; when lying down.*
BETTER *Stooping.*

HYPERICUM

CHARACTERISTICS

A great remedy for injuries to nerves.
Crushed fingers especially tips.
Excessive painfulness.
Punctured wounds.
Prevents lockjaw.

Head feels as though touched by an icy cold hand.
Throbbing vertex.
Head feels elongated.
Nausea.
Excellent for bleeding piles.
Pressure over sacrum.
Crawling in hands and feet.
Neuritis with tingling, burning pain.
Asthma worse foggy weather.
Wounded or punctured nerves; punctures from nails, splinters, pins etc., to severe concussion of spine and brain.
Consequences of spinal concussion.

"When finger ends or toes have been bruised or lacerated, or a nail torn off, or a nerve pinched between hammer and bone with a blow and that nerve becomes inflamed, and the pain can be traced to extending towards the body with stitching, darting pains or shooting up towards the body from the seat of the injury, a dangerous condition is coming on. Here Hypericum is above all remedies the one to be thought of . . . Lockjaw is threatening." – Kent.

MODALITIES
WORSE *In cold; dampness; fog; closed room; least exposure; touch.*
BETTER *Bending head backwards.*

IGNATIA

CHARACTERISTICS
A remedy of contradictions.
Mental stresses and strains from shock, bereavement, fright, etc.
Much grief; long sighs; sobbing; unhappiness.
Twitching, spasms or convulsions from depression, fright, emotion etc.
Great aversion to tobacco smoke.
Weak, empty sensation in stomach not relieved by eating.
Changeable moods. Nash says "Ignatia may justly be termed pre-eminently the remedy of MOODS."

Changeable moods.

Sighing and sobbing. Guernsey says "Anyone suffering from suppressed or deep grief, with long drawn sighs, much sobbing, also much unhappiness, can't sleep, entirely absorbed in grief; for recent grief, as at the loss of a friend; affections of the mind in general, particularly if actuated by grief; sadness; hopelessness; hysterical variableness; fantastic illusions."

Head worse stooping, feels hollow, heavy. Throbbing. Congestive headache worse smoking or smelling tobacco.

Weakness of sight.

Twitching of muscles of face and lips.

Sour taste in mouth.

Tonsils inflamed, swollen with small ulcers. Follicular tonsillitis.

Sensation of dry feathery dust in pit of throat not relieved by coughing.

Much flatulence in stomach. Sinking feeling better taking a deep breath.

Rectum prolapse.

Stools pass with difficulty; painful constriction of anus after stool.

Pressure as of a sharp instrument from within outward.

Menses black; too early, too profuse or scanty.

MODALITIES

WORSE *Morning; open air; after meals; coffee; smoking; external warmth*.

BETTER *While eating; change of position*.

IPECACUANHA

CHARACTERISTICS

Persistent nausea. Nausea unrelieved by vomiting.

Nausea and vomiting with clean tongue.

Haemorrhage bright red and profuse.

Peevish, irritable, impatient, scornful.

Ailments from vexation.

Nash summarizes Ipecacuanha as follows: "Persistent nausea, which nothing relieves, in many complaints.

"Headache as if bruised, all through the bones of the head, down to the root of tongue with nausea.

"Stools as if fermented, or as green as grass, with colic and nausea."

Haemorrhages from uterus; profuse, bright red, with nausea.

Spasmodic or asthmatic cough; great depression and wheezing; child becomes rigid and turns blue.

Backache, short chill, long fever, heat usually with thirst; raging headache, nausea; and sweats.

Ipecacuanha leads all the remedies for nausea.

With Ipecacuanha the tongue may be perfectly clean.

Sick headache with nausea.

Constant nausea and vomiting; much saliva in mouth.

Constriction of chest; cough incessant.

Whooping cough with nausea.

Slightest chill with heat, nausea and vomiting.

Old people with emphysema from chronic asthma benefit from Ipecacuanha.

MODALITIES

WORSE *Periodically; from veal; moist warm wind; lying down*.

KALI BICHROMICUM

CHARACTERISTICS

Discharge of tough, stringy, adherent mucus or jelly-like mucus
Pain comes in small spots.

"Kali Bichromicum is particularly adapted to fat, light-haired persons, or children disposed to catarrhal, croupy, scrofulous or syphilitic affections."
– Dr Drysdale who introduced this remedy.

Tough, stringy mucous discharges from eyes, ears, nose, mouth, throat, vomit, chest, urine, urethra and vulva.

Also jelly-like mucus from nose, posterior nares, vagina or anus and in stools of dysentary.

Pains appear and disappear suddenly.

Pain appears in spots the size covered by a finger-tip.

Ulcerations round and deep-looking as if they had been punched out.

Headache over eyebrows. Bones of scalp feel sore.

Discharge from eyes ropy and yellow.

Ears discharge thick, yellow, stringy foetid mucus.

Snuffles especially of fat, chubby babies.

Pressure and pain at root of nose. Septum ulcerated.

Discharge thick, ropy, greenish-yellow. Tough elastic plugs from nose. Loss of smell. Violent sneezing.

Tongue red, glazed, yellow, dry.

Round ulcer of stomach; vomiting ropy.

Dyspepsia. Feeling of weight and distress immediately after eating.

After urinating it feels as though a few drops remain and cannot be expelled.

Ropy, jelly-like leucorrhoea.

Hacking cough with profuse yellow, sticky expectoration coming away in long strings.

Rheumatism wandering, or alternating with catarrh or stomach troubles.

MODALITIES

WORSE *Beer, undressing; hot weather; 2 a.m.–3 a.m.*
BETTER *From heat.*

KALI CARBONICUM

CHARACTERISTICS

Very irritable.
Anxiety felt in stomach.
Fearful. Hates to be touched; and being alone.
Hypersensitive to pain, noise and touch.
All pains are sharp, cutting.
Stitches may be felt in any part of the body.
Intolerance of cold weather.

Anxiety felt in the stomach.

Great debility with weakened nerves. Sensitive and very easily frightened; cries out about imaginary appearances. Cannot bear to be touched. Hypersensitive to pain.

Headache from cold wind.

Swelling over upper eyelids like little bags. This is a very valuable symptom appearing with many affections.

Nose stuffs up in warm room. Ulcerated nostrils.

Sticking pain in throat.

Stomach distended, feels as if it would burst.

Much flatulence. Everything eaten turns to gas.

There is fullness, heat and great distention immediately after eating, even a little.

Abdomen distended after eating.

Anxiety felt in stomach.

Cough hard and dry with stitching pains worse around 3 a.m. Whole chest very sensitive.

Patient better sitting up and leaning forward, but worse lying on affected side. Very helpful for aged, ailing, anaemic people.

Small of back feels weak.

Pain in knees. Pain from hip to knee.

Soles of feet very sensitive.

MODALITIES

WORSE *After coition; in cold weather; from soup and coffee; about 3 a.m.; lying on left or painful side.*

BETTER *In warm moist weather, during the day; while moving about.*

KALI PHOSPHORICUM

CHARACTERISTICS

Prostration.
Want of nerve power.
Nervous dread.

One of the great nerve remedies.
    Prostration.
    Want of nerve power.
    Nervous dread.
    Night terrors.
    Slightest labour seems a heavy task.
    Brain fag. Has helped many children at end of term when they become languid and tired. Also overworked adults, especially those at office desks all day.
    Cerebral anaemia.
    Humming and buzzing in ears.
    Breath offensive; foetid.
    Extremely dry mouth, especially in the morning.
    Diarrhoea with foul, putrid odour.
    Menstruation too late and too scanty.
    Yellow urine.
    Yellow expectoration.

MODALITIES

WORSE *Excitement; worry; mental and physical exertion; eating; cold; early morning.*
BETTER *Warmth; rest; nourishment.*

LAC CANINUM

CHARACTERISTICS

Erratic pains, alternating sides.
Very fearful, especially of snakes and has visions of them.
Delusions and hallucinations.

This patient is very despondent, "there is nothing to live for" but carries on just the same!
    There is a fear of snakes, of falling, of disease, of death with anxiety.

Many delusions and hallucinations in daylight but not after dark; sees snakes and spiders; imagines all kinds of dreadful sights and is afraid they will be real. A sense of unreality is often present.

Forgetful; absent minded; irresolute.

Cracking of jaw while eating.

Throat symptoms change repeatedly.

Stiffness of neck and tongue.

Menses flow in gushes.

Breasts swollen; painful before but better as soon as menses appear.

Helps to dry up milk.

Never well since diphtheria.

MODALITIES

WORSE *Cold air; at night; after sleep; from movement; from touch. An aggravation may occur on alternate days or in the morning on one day and in the evening on the following day.*

BETTER *Warmth; when at rest; from lying down; in open air.*

LACHESIS

CHARACTERISTICS

Insanely jealous and suspicious.

Loquacity.

Worse from sleep. Sleeps into an aggravation (no matter what the symptoms).

Worse left side, sometimes moving to the right.

Intolerance of anything tight, especially round neck or waist.

Blueness anywhere points to Lachesis.

Tyler says "Lachesis affects supremely the throat and the mind."

Jealousy and suspicion are very marked in Lachesis; also loquacity, jumps from one subject to another.

Kent says "Self consciousness; self conceit; envy; hate and cruelty, an improper love of self; all sorts of impulsive insanity with purple face and head hot." are marked in this remedy.

"Quick comprehension with almost prophetic perception, ecstasy, a kind of trance." – Allen.

Weakness of memory. Confusion as to time.

Delirium at night. Sad; depressed.

Headaches when exposed to sun heat. Weight and pressure on top of head with pale face. Sleeps into headaches.

Intense suffering in throat quite out of proportion to anything that can be seen there. Choking sensations.

Feeling of constriction; Lachesis cannot bear throat to be touched and must have loose collars.

Tongue dry; trembles; puts it out with difficulty.

Throat symptoms worse hot drinks.

Serious throat conditions – ulcerations – diphtheria.

Swallowing solids more comfortable than empty swallowing.

Painful distention and flatulence worse pressure on stomach.

Painful and very difficult stools; anus feels closed; stools very offensive.

Asthma; cough during sleep.

Cough excited by touching throat.

Paroxysms of hayfever sneezing after sleep during the day.

MODALITIES

WORSE *After sleep (sleeps into an aggravation). Ailments that come on during sleep; left side; in the spring; warm bath; pressure or constriction; hot drinks; closing eyes.*

BETTER *Appearance of discharges; warm applications.*

LEDUM

CHARACTERISTICS

Rheumatism begins in the feet and travels upward.

Ecchymosis; black eye from a blow or contusion (better than Arnica).

Complaints of people who are cold all the time; lack of animal or vital heat; parts cold to touch, but not cold subjectively to patients.

Punctured wounds by sharp-pointed instruments, rat bites, stings of insects, especially mosquitoes.

Ledum has coldness relieved by cold.

Nash says "Ledum sometimes comes in to finish up an Arnica case; when Arnica was best at first Ledum often removes the ecchymoses (bruising) and discoloration more rapidly and perfectly." and "Black eye from a blow or contusion better than Arnica."

If a patient has a wound which feels cold, yet is ameliorated by cold applications Ledum will clear up the condition and deal with any tendency towards tetanus.

Ledum patients are discontented.

Noise in ears like bells ringing; roaring sound.

Painful respiration; constriction of chest.

Rheumatism begins in lower limbs and travels upwards but is most severe in lower parts. Worse warmth of bed.

Pains in shoulder joints.

Weakness in knee joints.

Abscesses and septic conditions; very tender; relieved by cold.

Puncture wounds from sharp, pointed instruments, awls, nails, rat bites, stings of insects etc., particularly if the wounded parts feel cold to touch and to patient.

Crushed fingers badly lacerated; throbbing, shooting up arm; relieved by cold; cured by Ledum.

MODALITIES

WORSE *At night; from heat of bed.*

BETTER *From cold; putting feet in cold water.*

LYCOPODIUM

CHARACTERISTICS

Intellectually keen but physically weak.

Upper part of body thin, lower part dropsical.

Very apprehensive – anticipation – before delivering address, lecture, etc., but fine as soon as she gets going.

Likes to be alone but somebody in the next room or other parts of the house.

Weeps when thanked.

Good appetite but a few mouthfuls fill up and she feels bloated.

Excessive accumulation of wind in lower abdomen.

Fullness – flatulence – distension.

Symptoms begin on right side and often move to the left.

Craves sweets.

Tyler says "Lycopodium has plenty of fears; fears of being alone; of crowds; of the dark; of death; of people."

Lycopodium has intellectual sufferings and failures and confusions when ill.

Melancholy; dislikes being alone; very apprehensive.

Spells or writes wrong words; irritable; peevish.

Dread of men. Weeps all day.

Easily angered, cannot bear opposition. Over sensitive to pain.

Ailments from fright, anger, vexation, mortification.

Headaches better uncovering.

Throbbing headache after coughing. Pain in temples as if screwed together, worse during menses.

Rush of blood to head on waking.

Night-blindness; styes of eyelids; ulceration and redness of eyelids.

Distressing pains as if eyes were dry.

Humming and roaring with hardness of hearing.

Eczema of ears with thick crusts and fissures.

Nose stopped up. Fan-like motion of alae nasi. Violent catarrh, cannot breathe at night. Complete stoppage of nose.

Tickling cough; chest feels oppressed and raw internally. Stitches in left side of chest when inspiring.

Blisters on tongue.

Inflammation of throat better warm drinks.

Ulceration of tonsils starting on right side. Deposits spread from right to left.

Food tastes sour.

Eating very little creates fullness.

Burning eructations rise to pharynx and burn for hours.

Abdomen bloated, full. Distention from gases.

Stool hard, difficult. Haemorrhoids very painful to touch, aching.

Urine slow in starting. Renal colic.

Impotence in male.

Burning between shoulder blades.

Sciatica worse right side. Cannot lie on painful side.

MODALITIES

WORSE *Right side; from right to left; from above downward; from 4 to 8 p.m.; (no other remedy has this as such an outstanding symptom); from heat or warm room; hot air, bed; warm applications except throat and stomach which are better from warm drinks.*

BETTER *By motion; after midnight; from warm food and drink; on getting cold, from being uncovered.*

MAGNESIA PHOSPHORICA

CHARACTERISTICS

The great anti-spasmodic remedy.
Neuralgia pains better by warmth.
Cramps.

Excruciating neuralgic or rheumatic headaches.

Severe neuralgic pains in ears worse washing face and neck in cold water.

Toothache better heat and hot liquids.

Complaints of teething children.

Throat puffy in parts with chilliness.

Pain in stomach with clean tongue.

Flatulent colic forcing patient to bend double, better rubbing, warmth and pressure; accompanied by belching of gas which gives no relief.

Bloated, full sensation in abdomen; must loosen clothing, walk about and constantly pass flatus.

Menstrual colic.

Dysmenorrhoea with violent abdominal pains which make patient double up; better by heat.

Spasmodic cough. Whooping cough.

Angina pectoris.

In fevers, chill runs up and down back with shivering followed by suffocating sensation.

Extremities. Chorea.

Tyler says "Nerve pains, then, with spasm, cramp and colic, suggest Mag. Phos. But one seems to notice that it is not indicated where there is fever – except in some fevers where there is cramp. The great sphere of the remedy is to torture, and to soothe, nerve tissue."

MODALITIES

WORSE *Right side; cold; touch; night*.
BETTER *Warmth; bending double; pressure; friction*.

MERCURIUS SOLUBIS

CHARACTERISTICS

Mouth offensive; tongue large, flabby, shows imprint of teeth.
Salivation with intense thirst.
Profuse perspiration which does not relieve.
Trembling; weakness.
All symptoms worse at night.
Sensitive to heat and cold.

Memory weak – forgets things.
    Hurried and rapid talking.

Mistrustful.

Whole head painful to touch. Congestion, feels it will burst; as if a band around head.

Catarrhal headaches; heat in head.

Mist before eyes; dimness of sight.

Dazzled by firelight. Lachrymation profuse, burning, excoriating. Discharges thin and acrid.

Aching in eyes; itching in eyeballs.

Roaring in ears. Inflammation internal and external; a feeling as if stopped up by swelling.

Nose bleed during sleep. Offensive odour from nose. Green, foetid pus. Nasal bone painful.

Corners of mouth ulcerated and sore. Teeth loose. Tongue white as if coated with fur. Swelling of tongue.

Gums swollen and painful.

Throat dry; constantly needs to swallow as mouth fills with water. Shooting pains on swallowing. Suppuration of tonsils with sharp, sticking pain when swallowing.

Salty taste in mouth; salt expectoration.

Taste of rotten eggs. Slimy taste.

Much water flows into mouth at night, wakens with nausea and vomits.

Hiccough.

Violent thirst.

Inguinal glands swollen, red, inflamed, painful.

Ineffectual urging to stool; bloody stools that excoriate anus; soft stools with burning pains. Green diarrhoea. Exhausted after stool.

Constant desire to urinate.

Greenish, biting leucorrhoea.

Frequent sneezing with coryza; stitches in chest with coughing.

Weakness of all limbs; hands tremble.

Perspiration profuse when walking; at night when it is also offensive and soaks bedclothes.

Large ulcers bleed.

Allen says "Merc. is worse by heat of bed but is better for rest in bed."

MODALITIES

WORSE *At night; warmth of bed; while sweating; lying on right side; damp weather.*

NATRUM CARBONICUM

CHARACTERISTICS

Great debility caused by summer heat.
Chronic effects of sunstroke.
Weakness of ankles.

This patient is greatly aggravated by mental exertion; headaches always develop when thinking, concentrating on some mental problem.

Gets very depressed; sad thoughts.

Great debility caused by summer heat.

Sensitive to noise; anxious and restless in thunder-storm.

Headaches from slightest mental exertion and in hot weather.

Chronic catarrh in nose which goes to posterior nares and throat; there is much hawking and spitting of thick mucus.

Very weak digestion caused by errors in diet.

Sudden call to stool, discharge yellow.

Weakness of ankles from childhood. Easy dislocation and sprains.

MODALITIES

WORSE *Sitting; from music; summer heat; mental exertion; thunder storm; least draught; changes of weather; sun.*
BETTER *By moving; by boring in ears and nose.*

NATRUM MURIATICUM

CHARACTERISTICS

Ill effects of grief, fright, anger.
Consolation aggravates; wants to be alone to cry.
Depressed; moody.
Very irritable.
Great weakness and weariness.
All mucous membranes dry.
Craves salt.
Very thirsty.

Natrum muriaticum is a deep acting, long lasting remedy. Kent says "It takes wonderful hold of the economy, making changes that are lasting. . . . It operates slowly, bringing about its results after a long time, as it corresponds to complaints that are slow and are long in action. This does not mean that it will not act rapidly; all remedies act rapidly but not all act slowly; the longest acting may act in acute cases but the shortest acting cannot in chronic disease."

Hurriedness with anxiety and fluttering heart. Depression. Sad, weeping moods without cause. Involuntary weeping. Consolation aggravates, patient hates it and becomes worse.

Tired of life. Indifferent.

Head dull, heavy. Pressing pain as if head would burst. Dandruff. Eyes weak; feeling of pressure. Muscles weak and stiff.

Violent, fluent coryza. Remember this remedy when colds commence with much sneezing.

Numbness of tongue; blisters; loss of taste; tongue mapped. Herpes around mouth. Unquenchable thirst.

Acid eructations. Sweats while eating. Craves salt.

Chronic diarrhoea, worse on moving about.

Constipation; unusually hard, crumbling stool.

Involuntary urination while walking, coughing, sneezing.

Intermittent heart beat especially when lying down.

Skin greasy; dry eruptions especially on margin of hair.

Fever with headache; chilliness; great thirst; with nausea and vomiting.

A remedy of periodicity.

Great emaciation even when living well.

MODALITIES
WORSE *Consolation; 10 a.m. to 11 a.m. (many complaints); lying down, especially on left side; heat, especially heat of sun; at seashore.*
BETTER *Open air; cold bathing; lying on right side; pressure against back.*

Natrum Sulphuricum

CHARACTERISTICS
Worse every spring.
Head symptoms from injuries to head.
Feels every change from dry to wet. Cannot tolerate sea air.
Aggravation of diarrhoea, pain etc., in damp weather.
Loose cough with soreness and pain through left chest.

Suicidal tendency, must exercise restraint; disturbed mind.

Depressed; irritable, worse mornings.

Pressure in forehead as if it would burst; better pressure. Heat on top of head. Brain feels loose when stooping.

After injury to head there may be violent pains especially at back of neck and base of brain.

Chronic conjunctivitis with granular lids, green pus, lids feel very heavy.

Nose stuffed up with dryness and burning. Catarrhal discharge yellow-green. Nose bleed before and/or after menses.

Palate sensitive, can hardly eat; relieved by anything cold.

Tongue burns as if covered with blisters.

Brown, bitter coating on tongue; bitter taste.

Thirst for something very cold.

Flatulent colic; flatus passed with difficulty. Cannot bear tight clothing round waist.

Vomiting of bile.

Tension and sticking pains in liver. Great sensitivity of liver, very painful when touched.

Loose morning stools; diarrhoea after rising; from vegetables, fruit, pastry, cold food and drink, and farinacous food.

Diarrhoea in wet weather.

Leucorrhoea yellowish-green.

Short breath with piercing pain in left side of chest.

Must hold chest when coughing. Pressure on chest. Oppression of chest.

Asthma in children.

Excruciating pain in right hip joint, worse stooping; when stretching or walking feels nothing. Pain in limbs, hands, fingers, worse moving in bed.

MODALITIES

WORSE *In the spring; warm, wet weather; dampness; 4–5 a.m.; any noise, even music.*
BETTER *Cool air; in dry weather.*

NITRIC ACID

CHARACTERISTICS

Has an affinity for mucous outlets; cracks, rhagades, fissures.
Pricking pains as if splinters were in the parts.
Urine strong smelling; like horse urine.
Haemorrhages from all outlets of body.
Pricking ulcers.

Irritable, dark complexioned people.

Depressed and very anxious in evening. Anxiety; despair; nervous, excitable; great weakness of memory.

Sensation of band round head. Vertigo on rising in morning.

Very sensitive to noise.

Sharp, sticking pains in eyes. Stitches in eyes. Smarting.

Roaring in ears; cracking when chewing. Deafness better when riding in vehicle.

Nosebleed. Corrosive discharge. Violent itching in nose. Ulceration of nostrils.

Corners of mouth cracked, ulcerated, scabby. Foul smell from mouth.

Tongue clean, red, wet with furrow in middle. Ulcers in soft palate with sharp, splinter-like pains. Ulcerated, spongy gums.

White patches on throat, ulcerated, swollen. Swallowing difficult. Stinging pains; sticking, painful sore throat.

Loves fat and salt. Bread disagrees. Jaundice. Pain in liver region.

Flatulence; rumbling in abdomen.

Anus cracked and fissured. Haemorrhoids protrude, crack, bleed, and very sore.

Pains after stool last for hours, even after soft stools.

Chronic diarrhoea.

Urine cold on passing; very offensive odour.

Shortness of breath going upstairs.

Cough, dry barking; tickling in larynx. Chronic dry, laryngeal cough with stinging and smarting.

Want of breath. Palpitation and anguish on going upstairs.

Panting.

Neuralgic pains in back.

Tearing in bones of lower extremities worse at night.

Great debility, heaviness and trembling of limbs worse at night.

Sweating at night.

MODALITIES

WORSE *Evening and night; cold and also hot weather*.
BETTER *When riding in a vehicle*.

NUX VOMICA

CHARACTERISTICS

Very irritable; fiery temperament; impatient; fastidious.
Can get excited, angry, spiteful and malicious.

Very particular and careful people.
Easily offended; anxious; depressed.
Sullen; fault-finding.
Over-sensitive to noise, slightest noise; strong odours; bright light; music.
Feels everything too strongly.
Quick in movement.
Very chilly and when unwell in spite of layers of clothing and hugging the
fire, still feels cold.

"Spasms; sensitiveness, chilliness; three general characteristics." – Nash.

Hering says "Oversensitiveness, every harmless word offends, every little noise frightens; anxious and beside themselves."

Nervous temperament. Excessive uneasiness.

Extreme sensitivity to least pain, least smell, noise or movement.

Quarrelsome, even to violence. Feels everything too strongly. Reproaches others for their faults. Sadness.

Intoxication. Drunken confusion of head.

Aching pain in occiput on waking; drunken giddiness of head in morning. Headache worse after eating with nausea and very sour vomiting.

Discharge from both nostrils obstructed by dry catarrh.

Coryza fluent during day, stopped at night.

Coryza with scraping in throat and much sneezing.

Throat rough with catarrh. Rawness in throat causing cough.

Cough from raw and scraped feeling in larynx.

Violent cough before rising in morning.

Scraping in chest causing hawking. Cough causes headache, as if skull would burst.

Asthma; tightness through chest on walking.

Shivering and chilliness on slightest movement or exposure to cold air.

Cannot get warm in spite of lots of clothing or bedcovers.

Putrid or bitter taste. Nausea in morning; after eating.

Nauseated and sick after a meal; pressure in stomach after eating a little.

Flatulent distension of abdomen. Colic causing nausea.

Blind haemorrhoids. Sharp pain in rectum after stool.

Feeling of something remaining in rectum after stool.

Frequent and ineffectual desire for stool, or passing small quantities at each attempt.

Frequent, painful, ineffectual desire to urinate.

Nausea in morning during menses.

Convulsions, twitching spasms of any muscles of the body, worse from slightest touch.

Lockjaw.

Menses early with cramps.

Backache low down, must sit up to turn over in bed.

MODALITIES

WORSE *Uncovering; mental work; after eating; cold air; dry weather; stimulants; 9 a.m.*

BETTER *Wet weather; warm room; on covering; after stool; from a nap, if allowed to finish it.*

OPIUM

CHARACTERISTICS

Fright; the fear of the fright remaining.

Complaints from fear.

Sleepy but cannot sleep; hears sounds not ordinarily noticed.

Abnormal painlessness.

Vivid imagination; exaltation of mind.

Fearful; expression of fright and terror.

Ailments from excessive joy, fright, anger, shame.

Spasms from emotion; fright.

Complete loss of consciousness.

Lightness of head in old people.

Very pale or flushed face. Face swollen, dark, suffused, hot.

Paralysis of tongue with difficult articulation.

Unquenchable thirst.

Colic violent, griping with constipation. Painter's colic.

Stools involuntary after fright; round, hard, black balls; fluid frothy; burning in anus. Almost incurable constipation.

Retention of urine but involuntary after fright.

Respirations long, sighing; deep snoring; rattling stertorous breathing.

Pulse full and slow in fevers.

Hot, perspiring skin over whole body except lower limbs.

"Painlessness in all ailments, complains of nothing; wants nothing." – Nash.

MODALITIES
WORSE *Heat; during and after sleep*.
BETTER *Cold things; constant walking*.

PETROLEUM

CHARACTERISTICS
Long lasting complaints follow mental states; fright; vexations.
Marked aggravation from mental emotions.
Seasickness.
Diarrhoea preceded by colic only in daytime.
Skin eruptions, all worse in winter, better in summer.

Irritable, quarrelsome; delirium. Forgetful, not disposed to think. Patient thinks death is near, he must hurry to settle his affairs. Very miserable and depressed.

Head sensitive as if a cold breeze is blowing on it. Moist eruption on scalp.

Vertigo on rising.

Headache in occiput which feels very heavy.

Great pressure in eyes. Lids red, inflamed, covered with scabs.

Whizzing, roaring and cracking in ears with reduced hearing.

Redness and soreness behind ears.

Nostrils ulcerated, cracked, burning.

Nausea every morning after waking; cannot eat breakfast.

Accumulation of water in mouth, suddenly with nausea.

Seasickness.

After slight meal feels giddy; nausea all day.

Hoarseness; cough from dryness in throat.

Sharp pains going up spine to back of head.

Diarrhoea only in daytime; hunger after stool.

Skin cracked, rough, bleeding, dry, sensitive; leathery.

Painful chilblains on hands. Tips of fingers rough, cracked, fissured.

"Eczemas on scalp, behind ears, scrotum, anus, hands, feet, legs. Hands chap and bleed. All worse in winter; get better in summer." – Nash.

MODALITIES
WORSE *Damp; in winter; before and during thunderstorms; riding in vehicles; from mental states.*
BETTER *Warm air; dry weather.*

PHOSPHORIC ACID

CHARACTERISTICS

Drowsy, apathetic, unconscious but can be aroused to full consciousness.
Grows too fast and too tall.
Great physical and mental weakness.
Depression.
Pinching and squeezing pains.

The remedy for ailments from grief, chagrin, home-sickness, disappointed love.

Listless; apathetic; indifferent. Cannot collect thoughts.

Mind tired; nerve strain.

Guernsey says ". . . a condition of complete indifference to everything; not a soporous, delirious or irritable condition but simply an indifferent state of mind to all things. He does not want anything, nor to speak; shows no interest in the outside world."

Nash says "The profound weakness and depression of Phos. acid is upon the sensorium and nervous system."

Occipital headaches and pains in nape of neck from exhausted nerve power or grief.

Confusion of head; buzzing in head.

Tearing pains; sensations of squeezing and pressure in various parts of head.

Pain from pressure in eyeballs.

Dry feeling in mouth with nausea.

Great thirst for cold milk.

Pressure in stomach after eating. Rumbling in abdomen.

White or yellow watery diarrhoea without pain or debility.

Stools involuntary.

Urging but scanty discharge of urine.

Pale urine which soon forms a thick, whitish cloud.

Great hoarseness. Difficult inspiration; pain in chest from weakness.

Hips, thighs, arms and nape feel bruised.

Exhaustion in legs when walking.

Feeling of ants running about. Itching in body and hands.

Can hardly be wakened from sleep in the morning.

Inflammation of bones; feeling as if bone were scraped with a knife.

Growing pains.

This remedy helps weedy, overgrown teenagers.

MODALITIES

WORSE *Exertion; from being talked to; loss of vital fluids; symptoms from impeded circulation.*

BETTER *After a short sleep; from warmth.*

PHOSPHORUS

CHARACTERISTICS

Extremely sensitive.

Fearful of thunderstorms; being alone; of the dark; disease; death.

Very affectionate; they need it and give it, yet there can be an indifference.

Desire to be rubbed.

Patient moves continually; cannot stand or sit still.

Much weakness and trembling.

Burning; heat in various parts, particularly the skin.

Haemorrhages bright and freely flowing.

Thirst for cold drinks which are vomited as soon as they become warm.

Nash says "The person who needs Phos. is tall, slender, narrow chested, phthisical, with delicate eyelashes, soft hair; or nervous weak persons who like to be magnetised." He added "Phos. is fidgety all over; is bound to bleed and it attacks the bones in the form of necrosis."

Apathy; sluggishness. Talks slowly or not at all. Hates to be left alone; fears something will happen.

Very indifferent. Is sympathetic, craves company and touch. Anxious; cannot stand or sit still.

Hypersensitive. Anxious at twilight; fear of thunder. Full of strange imaginations. Worse from manual exertion.

Prostration; trembling; numbness.

Vertigo on rising.

Photophobia.

Bloating around eyes.

Deafness, especially to human voice.

Nose-bleed.

Vomiting of food. Pressure in stomach.

"Craves cold things; ice-cream which agrees, cold water which may be vomited when it gets to the stomach. Must eat often or is faint. Gets up to eat in the night. Sinking, faint, empty feelings everywhere." – Nash.

Sensation of weakness and emptiness in abdomen.

Rawness of larynx with frequent hacking cough.

Husky voice.

Cough which hurts chest. Violent dry cough when talking a lot.

Cough from constant tickling of throat and difficult respiration.

Bloody expectoration with mucus, and from lungs.

Respiration anxious and difficult; laboured.

Patient must sit up in bed; distressing anxiety and pressure in chest.

Anxiety around heart. Violent palpitation.

Burning pains between shoulders. Weakness of all limbs.

Constant sleepiness even during the day.

Heat at night without thirst.

Profuse sweats every morning and on slight exertion.

"Unable to drink water during pregnancy; sight of water makes her vomit; must close eyes while bathing." – Allen.

"Phos. is the surgeon's friend – the great remedy for vomiting after chloroform." – Nash.

MODALITIES

WORSE *Touch; physical or mental exertion; twilight; warm food or drink; from getting wet in hot weather; evening; lying on left or painful side; during thunder storms.*

BETTER *In the dark; lying on right side; cold food; cold; open air; washing with cold water; sleep.*

PHYTOLACCA

CHARACTERISTICS

Pre-eminently a glandular remedy.

Aching; soreness; restlessness; prostration.

Irresistible inclination to bite teeth or gums together.

Hale says "Phytolacca affects the nervous system also the fibrous and osseous tissues."

Intense headache. Painful pressure on forehead and upper part of both eyes.

Smarting eyes with much lachrymation.

Mucus from one nostril and from posterior nares.

Face flushed.

Red tip of tongue.

Throat dark or bluish red; feels rough, narrow and hot.

Tonsils swollen followed by white spots; shooting pains into ears on swallowing.

Throat burning; cannot swallow anything hot; pain at root of tongue extending to ear.

Urine suppressed with pain in kidney region.

Mastitis, breasts hard and sensitive. When child is breast-fed pain goes from nipple all over body.

Abscesses or fistular ulcers of breasts.

Mammary gland full of hard, painful nodes.

Nipples cracked and excoriated.

Rheumatic pains worse morning. Pains fly like electric shocks, shifting rapidly. Aching of heels.

In sciatica pains run down outer side of limbs.

Disposition to boils.

High fever, pulse quick, but heat mostly in head and face while body and limbs are cool.

MODALITIES

WORSE *When it rains; exposure to damp; cold weather; in cold room; night; motion; right side.*

BETTER *Warmth; dry weather; rest.*

PLUMBUM

- -

CHARACTERISTICS

Abdomen retracted to spine as if drawn in by a string.

Distinct blue line along margin of gums.

Wrist-drop; paralysis of extensor muscles.

Progressive muscular atrophy.

Excessive and rapid emaciation.

A very important indication from Nash is "Hyperaesthesia with loss of power."

Mental depression. Slow perception. Hallucinations and delusions. Kent says "Plumbum is intensely emotional while the intellect is slowed down."

Pain as if ball rose from throat to brain.

Constriction of throat.

Whites of eyes very yellow. Optic nerve inflamed.

Face very pale; skin greasy, shiny and yellow.

Distinct blue line along margin of gums. Tongue tremulous, feels paralysed.

Contraction in oesophagus and stomach. Constant vomiting. Loss of appetite. Nausea.

Colic in abdomen radiating to all parts of body.

Abdominal wall feels drawn up by a string to spine.

Abdomen retracted. Obstructed flatus with painful colic.

Stools hard, lumpy, black with urging and spasm of anus.

Anus drawn up with constriction.

Chronic nephritis. There is increase of mucus in urine with irritation of the lining membrane of bladder.

Loss of sexual power in male.

Vaginismus. Induration of mammary glands.

Yellow, dark brown liver spots.

Paralysis of single muscles. Wrist-drop.

Pain in big right toe at night.

Violent and/or neuralgic pains in extremities.

Jerking, trembling, numbness of limbs.

MODALITIES

WORSE *At night; motion.*

BETTER *Rubbing; hard pressure; physical exertion.*

PODOPHYLLUM

CHARACTERISTICS

Suited to persons of bilious temperament.

Loquacity.

Depression.

Worse in hot weather.

Adapted to people of bilious temperament.

Many troubles during pregnancy.

Loquacity. Depression.

Headache alternating with diarrhoea. Rolling of head from side to side with moaning and vomiting.

Great desire to press the gums together. Tongue broad, large, moist. Burning sensation.

Sensation of sinking and weakness of abdomen.

Pains around liver, better by rubbing.

Diarrhoea, early morning; in children when teething with hot, glowing cheeks. Green, watery, foetid, profuse, gushing stools. Prolapse of rectum before or with stool.

Pain in uterus and right ovary with noises passing along ascending colon. Prolapsed uterus.

Jaundice.

Haemorrhoids with prolapse during pregnancy.

MODALITIES

WORSE *Early morning; in hot weather; during dentition.*

PULSATILLA

CHARACTERISTICS

The temperament is mild and gentle but anger can appear, and irritability.

Tears come very easily; inclined to silent grief.

Conscientious, hates to be hussled.

Loves sympathy and fuss.

Changeable in everything; in disposition (like an April shower and sunshine); pains wander from joint to joint; no two stools are alike, etc.

Pulsatilla feels the heat; they must have air, it makes them feel much better.

Cannot eat fat, rich food, it makes them feel sick.

Thirstless, even with a fever.

Hahnemann says "Pulsatilla is especially adapted for slow, phlegmatic temperaments; and little suited for persons who form their resolutions with rapidity, and are quick in their movements, even though they may appear to be good tempered."

Mild, gentle disposition. Sad and despondent.

Weeps easily. Timid; irresolute.

Symptoms always changing.

Vertigo as from intoxication. Vertigo especially when sitting.

Neuralgic pains. Headache from overwork. Heaviness in head.

Thick, profuse, yellow, bland discharges from eyes. Lids inflamed, agglutinated. Styes on lids. Itching and burning which compels rubbing of eyes.

Nosebleed with stuffy coryza.

Bad taste in mouth, worse mornings, with great dryness but no thirst. Crack in middle of lower lip.

Pressing pain at root of nose. Yellow mucus.

Yellow or white tongue covered with tenacious mucus.

Taste bitter, greasy, salty, foul, and as if burnt.

Throat painful, sore, scratchy, dry.

Stomach easily disturbed, especially by cakes, pastry or rich, fat foods. Averse to fat food, warm food and drink.

Much sweet saliva. Diminished taste of all food.

Flatulence. Frequent eructations.

Sensation of sickness in epigastric region. Inclination to vomit.

Flatulent colic immediately after supper.

Flatus discharged with cutting pain in abdomen in morning.

Stomach ache after stool. Frequent urging. Stools of yellow-white mucus.

Frequent urination. Urine dribbles when sitting or walking.

Menses dark, clotted, changeable.

Acute prostatitis.

Dry cough in evening and at night, must sit up in bed. Loose cough in morning. Pressure and soreness of chest.

Chilliness of extremities. Pain changing rapidly.

Chilliness in fevers without thirst. External heat intolerable, veins become distended.

Palpitation with great anxiety.

Wakens from sleep frightened and confused.

Moves about in sleep.

MODALITIES

WORSE *Heat; rich, fat food; after eating; warmth; in warm room; towards evening.*

BETTER *In open cold air and from cold applications; cold food and drinks though not thirsty.*

RHUS TOXICODENDRON

CHARACTERISTICS

Extreme restlessness with continued change of position.
Great apprehension at night.
Cannot remain in bed.
Triangular red tip of tongue.

Hahnemann says "The severest symptoms and sufferings are excited when the body or limb is at rest and kept as much as possible without movement."

Kent says of Rhus "He is never properly at ease and never finds rest."

But Guernesy explains clearly "We are led to think of this remedy when we find an irresistible desire to move, or change the position every little while, followed by great relief for a short time, when they must again move and again experience the same relief for a short time. After resting, when first moving a painful stiffness is felt which wears off from continued motion."

Sad; weeps without knowing why. Very restless.

Great apprehension at night; cannot remain in bed.

Giddy on rising.

Inflammation of eyes; very swollen lids; red and agglutinated. Lids heavy and stiff, opening eyes difficult.

Frequent, violent, spasmodic sneezing. Much mucus from nose.

Yawning violent and spasmodic.

Tongue sore, dry.

Throat swollen externally; glands enlarged.

Great thirst with dryness of throat.

Cough from severe tickling and irritation behind sternum.

Stiffness in small of back; also heaviness and pressure.

Limbs stiff on first moving after rest. Aching and restlessness in all limbs.

Pressing pain in hip-joint. Stiffness and tension in knees.

Weakness of limbs.

Erysipelas.

Red, vesicular rash over body; burning, itching; no relief from scratching. Skin burning; hot.

Urticaria; worse in cold air.

Eczema; raw, excoriated; thick crusts; oozing, offensive.

Burning, itching, tingling pains.

Slow fevers; great weakness; lower limbs powerless.

Great restlessness midnight.

MODALITIES

WORSE *Damp and cold; wet, rainy weather; after rain; at night; during rest; lying on back or right side.*

BETTER *Warm, dry weather; motion; walking; change of position; rubbing; warm applications; from stretching limbs.*

RUTA

CHARACTERISTICS

Acts upon the periosteum and cartilages.
Complaints from straining flexor tendons especially.
All parts of body are painful as if bruised.

Feeling of intense weakness, lassitude and despair.

Shooting pains in head; pain as if from a fall.

Sensation of heat and fire in eyes; eyes feel tired after reading too much. Aching in and over eyes, with blurred vision after using them too much. Vision weak. Itching on lower lids. Spasm in lower eyelid; sensation as though a blunt object had been pushed into it.

Cartilages and under mastoid process pains as from a blow or fall.

Tension in stomach, better drinking milk.

Aching pain in hepatic region.

Tearing stitches in rectum when sitting.

Gnawing left side of chest.

Pain as if beaten in spine, worse when sitting.

Pain in elbow joint as from blow with weakness.

Bones of wrist and back of hand painful as if bruised.

Cannot bend body. All joints and hips painful as if bruised.

Difficulty going up and down stairs; legs bend under.

Bones of feet painful.

Very restless legs.

Lameness after sprains, especially of wrists and ankles.

All parts lain on in bed painful as if bruised.

Bruises and mechanical injuries of bones and periosteum; sprains; periostitis; erysipelas.

The pains of Ruta are generally from weariness rather than from weakness.

MODALITIES

WORSE *From cold and wet; lying on painful side; when at rest; when walking out of doors; by touch; from stooping.*

BETTER *By motion; warmth.*

SEPIA

CHARACTERISTICS

Great indifference to family (to husband and often children) and friends.

Averse to work; loses interest in what she ordinarily loves.

Irritable.

Easily offended.

Anxious.

Dreads to be alone.

Nervous; jumpy; hysterical.

Weeps when telling symptoms.

Depressed.
Hates sympathy and weeps if it is offered.
Wants to get away to be quiet.
Weakness; weariness.
Pains travel upwards.
A "ball" sensation in inner parts.
Faints when kneeling.
Feels the cold, must have air.
Gnawing hunger.
Craves vinegar and sour things.
Aversion to meat, fat and often bread and milk.

Kent says "Sepia is suited to tall, slim women with narrow pelvis and lax fibres and muscles. . . . one of the strongest features of the Sepia patient is found in the mind, the state of the affections. . . . the remedy seems to abolish the ability to feel natural love, to be affectionate. . . . 'I know I ought to love my children and my husband, I used to love them but now I have no feeling on the subject'. . . . the love does not go forth into affection. . . . an absence of all joy, inability to realize things are real. . . ."

Great irritability; very indifferent, apathetic; lacking in enthusiasm and zest for anything.

A desire to escape yet a dread of complete solitude; a tendency to restlessness, frustration and sometimes arguments. Symptoms from over-work, strain and fear; a broken down constitution, yet deep down there is determination and desire to get well.

Headache, right sided with surging sensation; waves of pain against frontal bone. Tearing in left temple.

Headache every morning with nausea, vertigo, nosebleed; with a feeling of emptiness in stomach and aversion to many foods. Headache better after meals.

Smarting of right eye; lids close involuntarily; sensation of sand in eyes, especially right.

Face pale; yellowness of face and whites of eyes.

Yellow saddle across bridge of nose.

Nostrils sore, swollen, ulcerated and scabby; discharge of large green plugs.

Nausea in morning better eating.

Faint, sinking, empty feeling in stomach.

Nausea after eating; from smell of cooking; riding in a vehicle.

Morning sickness of pregnancy. Burning in pit of stomach.

Bearing down sensation in pelvic organs.

Distension, rumbling or sensation of emptiness in abdomen.

Pressure in abdomen as though contents would drop through genital organs.

Pressure in uterus as though contents would go through vulva.

Constipation during pregnancy.

Prolapse of uterus, of vagina, with constipation.

Before menses acrid leucorrhoea.

Hot flushes at climacteric with sweat, weakness and faintness.

Spasmodic cough; cannot sleep for incessant cough.

When stooping sudden pain in back as though it had been struck.

Sudden prostration; faintness when kneeling.

Flushes of heat. Profuse night sweats and from least exertion.

Chilly patients but they feel faint in hot, stuffy rooms.

MODALITIES

WORSE *In dull, cloudy weather; before thunderstorms; sitting still; before menses; late morning; at dusk; washing; dampness.*

BETTER *Brisk exercise, especially in open air (if energy will allow); walking against wind; warmth of bed; food; after sleep; hard pressure and during afternoon.*

SILICA

CHARACTERISTICS

Want of grit – moral and physical.

Yielding; faint hearted; anxious.

Very sensitive to all impressions.

Easily irritated over trifles; touch; self-willed.

Fixed ideas.

Intolerance of alcohol.

Suppurative processes.

Under nourished from imperfect assimilation.

Feels the cold.

A French paediatrician described a typical Silica child as follows: "The little Silica patient is full of apprehension. He lacks confidence in himself and always thinks that he will be incapable of writing a composition or learning a lesson. The Silica subject's lack of confidence plays it's part in the difficulty he has in fixing his attention. He is too tired to stick to a task which he is too timid to undertake. With his back to the wall he can get annoyed, can grumble and can get angry."

Dr Vannier says "Silica is the remedy of depth for the overworked individual whose nervous resistance is used up."

Great difficulty in fixing his attention. Thinking difficult. Weariness and weakness. Internal restlessness and excitement.

Violent headache rising from nape of neck. Feeling as if head would burst. Pressive pain in occiput relieved by wrapping head up warmly. Profuse sweat on head.

Ears sensitive to loud sounds.

Gums painfully sensitive to cold water.

Abdomen hard, tense. Offensive flatus.

Haemorrhoids painfully sensitive. Stool remains long in rectum.

Burning in anus after hard, dry stool.

Stools can be very hard, difficult and after protruding may slip back again.

Right breast hard, painful, swollen at nipple. If child nurses it vomits; aversion to mother's milk.

Weakness of all limbs.

Offensive perspiration on the feet.

Boils on different parts of the body. Unhealthy skin, every little injury suppurates.

Restless sleep.

Chilly on every movement. Icy cold feet in evening and in bed preventing sleep; during menses.

Fever with violent heat in head.

Profuse perspiration every night towards morning.

Most of Silica's symptoms occur at the new moon.

MODALITIES

WORSE *Cold air; in cold weather; change from damp to dry weather; before and during thunderstorms; draughts; from pressure; during menstrual period; at new and full moon; lying on left side.*
BETTER *When warmly wrapped up, especially head; by hot applications; in summer; when lying down.*

SPIGELIA

CHARACTERISTICS

Violent beating of the heart, sometimes audible several inches away.
Neuralgias, pains increase and decrease with the rising and setting sun.
Very sensitive to touch.

Nash says "In this we have another invaluable heart remedy. . . . it is one of our best remedies for neuralgic affections of the head, face and eyes."

Afraid of sharp, pointed things – pins, needles etc.

Headaches one-sided, beginning at back of head, extending forward and settling over left eye. They increase with rising and decrease with setting of sun. Eye affected often runs clear water.

Pressive pain on turning eyes. Severe pain in and around eyes extending into sockets.

Chronic catarrh.

Foul odour from mouth.

Violent palpitation; patient can lie only on right side or with head very high; shortness of breath.

Neuralgia extending to one or both arms.

MODALITIES

WORSE *From motion; noise; moving eyes; cold, damp, rainy weather.*
BETTER *Quiet; dry air; setting sun.*

SPONGIA

CHARACTERISTICS

Croupy cough, sounds like a saw driven through a board; worse on waking.
Exhaustion and heaviness of body after slight exertion.
Wakens from sleep from a sense of suffocation with violent, loud cough, great alarm, agitation and difficult respiration.

Anxiety and fear, with difficult breathing.

Can have great hunger.

Palpitation before menses. During menses wakes up with suffocative spells.

Hoarseness; larynx dry, burning.

Cough dry, barking, croupy; croup worse when inspiring and before midnight.

Respiration difficult, feeling as of a plug in larynx. Cough better after eating or drinking; worse talking, singing, swallowing.

Awakened suddenly, after midnight with pain and suffocation.

Surging of heart to chest.

Waking from sleep feeling frightened and as if suffocating.

In fever attacks of heat with anxiety.

MODALITIES

WORSE *Ascending; in wind; before midnight.*
BETTER *Descending.*

STAPHISAGRIA

CHARACTERISTICS

Complaints from pent-up wrath; suppressed anger and feelings.
Very sensitive.
Severe pain following abdominal operation.
Irritable bladder in young married women.
Scratching changes location of itching.
Backache, worse in morning before rising.

Violent outbursts of passion.

Very sensitive as to what is said about her.

Weakness of memory, cannot remember what he has read. Indifference; dullness of mind.

Anger or indignation from least word or action that annoys or troubles him.

Aching, stupifying pain in head.

Recurrent styes on lids and scurfy margins of eyelids.

Inflammation of white of eye with pains.

Tearing stitch in left ear.

Stitches flying from throat to ear on swallowing, especially left.

Teeth black and crumbling. Much toothache, worse cold drinks and touch.

Craving for tobacco.

Extreme hunger even when stomach is full of food.

Sensation as if stomach and abdomen were hanging down.

Much hot flatus is developed.

Shivering and chilly feeling when eating without thirst.

Irritable bladder in young married women.

Ineffectual urging to urinate in newly married women.

Sensation of urine left behind.

Frequent call to urinate but little is passed.

Eczema, dry and itching; scratching changes location of itching.

Backache, worse morning before rising; and at night in bed.

Crural neuralgia.

For clean cut wounds, as after surgical operations.

MODALITIES

WORSE *Anger; indignation; grief; mortification; loss of fluids; sexual excesses; tobacco; least touch on affected parts.*
BETTER *After breakfast; warmth; rest; at night.*

STRAMONIUM

CHARACTERISTICS

Wildly delirious with red face and great loquacity.
Loquacity.
Wants light and company; fears to be alone.
One side paralyzed, the other convulsed.
Awakens frightened.
Painlessness with most complaints.

Boger says of Stramonium "A remedy of terrors but lacking in pain. . . . dreads darkness and has a horror of glistening objects. . . . great thirst but dreads water. . . . putrid, dark painless, involuntary diarrhoea. . . . awakes in fear screaming."

Noisy delirium with hallucinations.

Great stupidity.

Violence; excitement; rage. Anxious; fearful.

Mind in an uproar.

Symptoms resembling hydrophobia.

Irrational.

Jerks head frequently from pillow.

Head very hot.

Eyes stare, wide open; pupils dilated. Complains of darkness, wants light.

Small objects look large.

Expression of terror on face. Face hot and red.

Mouth and throat dry.

Stammers.

Violent thirst. Vomits mucus and green bile.

Glairy saliva dribbling from mouth.

Constriction of throat with kind of paralysis.

Abdomen distended; stool and urine suppressed.

Twitchings, of hands and feet, through body like chorea.

Trembling; convulsions.

Constant restless movements of all limbs and whole body.

Skin hot, dry, burning, scarlet.

Wakes from sleep terrified; screams.

Effects of suppressed eruptions.

There is an entire absence of pain.

MODALITIES

WORSE *In dark room; when alone; looking at bright or shining objects; after sleep.*
BETTER *From bright light; company; warmth.*

SULPHUR

CHARACTERISTICS

This remedy is known as the ragged philosopher.
Selfish, lazy and untidy people who often fling themselves into a chair with one leg draped over an arm.
Philosophical people wanting to know the "Why's and wherefore's."
Skin burning and itching, worse from warmth of bed.
Red orifices; eyes, nose, ears, lips and anus.
Sinking feeling mid-morning.
Worse standing.
Discharges offensive; acrid and excoriating, making part over which they flow red and burning.
Dislike of water; of washing.
Cat-nap sleep.

"Sulphur is one of the greatest of 'polycrests' (drugs of many uses) – is Hahnemann's Prince of 'antipsorics' (remedies of non-venereal chronic diseases) – and is one of the constituents of protoplasm, thus not only occurring, but evoking and curing symptoms in every tissue and organ of the body." – Tyler.

Foolish happiness and pride.

Indisposed to everything; indolence of mind and body.

Melancholy; anxiety; indifference; lazy.

Constant heat on top of head.

Scalp dry, itching; scratching causes burning.

Burning ulceration of eye-lids and in eyes.

Chronic dry catarrh; nose scabby and bleeding. Lips bright red and burning.

Bitter taste in mouth.

Great acidity in stomach with sour eructations; milk disagrees. Feels weak and faint around 11 a.m., must eat something.

Redness around anus. Morning diarrhoea which is painless but drives patient out of bed.

Bed wetting; mucus and pus in urine, parts sore over which it passes. Sudden call to urinate.

Vagina burns. Menses late, short and scanty; thick, black and acrid making parts sore.

Difficult breathing, wants air. Much rattling of mucus. Oppression as of a load on chest. Breathless in night, better sitting up.

Pulse rapid in morning.

Hot, sweaty hands. Burning in soles of feet and hands at night.

Stoop shouldered.

Catnaps.

Frequent flushes of heat in fever.

Dry, scaly, unhealthy skin; every little injury suppurates.

Itching; burning; worse scratching and washing.

Pruritis.

MODALITIES

WORSE *At rest; standing; warmth of bed; washing; around 11 a.m.; from alcoholic stimulants.*

BETTER *Dry, warm weather; lying on right side; from drawing up affected limbs.*

THUJA

CHARACTERISTICS

Ill effects of vaccination.
Rapid exhaustion and emaciation.
Sweats only on uncovered parts.
Antidote to tea.

Apathetic, wants to be left alone. Feels dazed, confused, especially on waking.

Peevish; great sensitivity to people, atmosphere, music.

Fixed ideas; as if something alive in abdomen; thinks legs are made of wood.

Emotional sensitiveness.

Neuralgia; headache as if pierced by nail.

Nervous, sycotic or syphilitic headaches.

Chronic catarrh, thick, green mucus. Ulceration in nostrils.

Painful pressure at root of nose.

White blisters on side of mouth, very sore.

Flatulence and distension of abdomen.

Gonorrhoeal rheumatism in men.

Prostatic affections from suppressed gonorrhoea.

Anus fissured, painful, often with warts.

Warts. Eruptions only on covered parts of skin. Cauliflower excrescences smelling like old cheese or herring brine.

Brown spots on hands and arms.

Joints crack; limbs jerk; muscles feel as if beaten; stiffness and heaviness felt all over.

Sleeplessness; parts lain on painful; from heat, restlessness, mental depression; sees apparitions on closing eyes.

All symptoms tend to be severe and excessive but their onset is insidious.

Pains shooting, burning, darting; may drive him out of bed.

Flushes of heat and pulsations, especially in evening.

Discharges profuse.

A left-sided remedy.

MODALITIES

WORSE *Damp, cold weather; heat of bed; bright light and direct sun; movement; drinking tea or coffee; taking narcotics; during menstrual period; at night; after breakfast; at 3 a.m. and 3 p.m.*
BETTER *Cool air; after sweating; by stretching limbs; from scratching; being massaged.*

VERATRUM ALBUM

CHARACTERISTICS

Collapse with general coldness; cold sweat especially on forehead.
Mania with desire to cut and tear things; with lewd lascivious, religious or amorous talk.
If irritated becomes mad, otherwise silent.
Cold perspiration on forehead with nearly all complaints.
Profuse, violent retching and vomiting.

Sullen indifference.

Delusions of impending misfortunes.

Cold sweat on forehead; sensation of lump of ice on vertex.

Icy coldness of tip of nose and face. Face pale, blue, collapsed, cold.

Voracious appetite. Thirst for cold water which is vomited as soon as swallowed. Much vomiting and nausea worse from drinking and any motion.

Cold feeling in stomach and abdomen.

Stools large; much straining exhausts, with cold sweat.

Dysmenorrhoea with coldness and cold sweat. Faints from least exertion.

Cramps in calves.

Rheumatism worse in wet weather; pains drive patient out of bed.

Skin blue, cold, clammy; cold as death.

Chill with extreme coldness.

"Rapid sinking of forces; complete prostration; cold sweat and cold breath; skin blue, purple, cold, wrinkled, remaining in folds when pinched. Face hippocratic; nose pointed; whole body icy cold. Cold skin, face cold, back cold. Hands icy cold. Feet and legs icy cold. Cramps of calves." – Nash.

MODALITIES

WORSE *At night; wet, cold weather*.
BETTER *Walking; warmth*.

ZINCUM METALLICUM

CHARACTERISTICS

Period of depression in disease.
Convulsions with pale face and no heat.
Fidgety feet, must move them constantly.
Twitching of single muscles all over body.
Violent trembling all over.

Nervous debility; lethargic; stupid.

Very sensitive to noise.

Pain in back of hand with sensation of weight on top.

Forehead cool; base of brain feels hot.

Rolling of eyes. Squinting.

Aching and weariness in nape of neck, from any exertion.

Smallest quantity of wine upsets.

Ravenous hunger around 11 a.m.

Griping after eating.

Cholera infantum.

Ovarian pain, especially left; cannot stay still.

All complaints better during menstrual flow.

Female complaints are associated with restlessness, depression, coldness, spinal tenderness and restless feet.

Asthmatic bronchitis; shortness of breath better as soon as patient brings up mucus.

Dull aching in back, worse sitting. Burning along spine.

Weakness, tremblings and twitchings. Feet in constant motion. Large varicose veins on legs.

Soles of feet sensitive.

MODALITIES

WORSE *At menstrual period; from touch; between 5 to 7 p.m.; from wine; after dinner.*

BETTER *Eating; discharges; appearance of eruptions.*

REPERTORY

ABBREVIATIONS

ACONITUM NAPELLUS .... Acon.

AGARICUS MUSCARIUS .... Agar.

ALLIUM CEPA .... All.c.

ALUMINA .... Alum.

AMBRA GRISEA .... Amb.g.

AMMONIUM CARBONICUM .... Amm.c.

AMMONIUM MURIATICUM .... Amm.m.

ANACARDIUM .... Anac.

ANTIMONIUM CRUDUM .... Ant.c.

ANTIMONIUM TARTARICUM .... Ant.t.

APIS MELLIFICA .... Apis.

ARGENTUM NITRICUM .... Arg.n.

ARNICA MONTANA .... Arn.

ARSENICUM ALBUM .... Ars.

AURUM METALLICUM .... Aur.

BAPTISIA .... Bapt.

BARYTA CARBONICA .... Bar.c.

BELLADONNA .... Bell.

BERBERIS .... Berb.

BORAX .... Bor.

BRYONIA .... Bry.

CACTUS GRANDIFLORA .... Cact.

CALCAREA CARBONICA .... Calc.c.

CALCAREA PHOSPHORICA .... Calc.p.

CALENDULA .... Calen.

CANTHARIS .... Canth.

CARBO VEGETABILIS .... Carb.v.

CAUSTICUM .... Caust.

CHAMOMILLA .... Cham.

CHELIDONIUM .... Chel.

CIMICIFUGA .... Cimic.

CINCHONA OFFICINALIS (CHINA) .... China.

COCCULUS INDICA .... Cocc.

COFFEA .... Coff.

COLCHICUM .... Colch.

COLOCYNTHIS .... Colo.

CUPRUM METALLICUM .... Cup.m.

DROSERA .... Dros.

DULCAMARA .... Dulc.

FERRUM METALLICUM .... Ferr.m.

GELSEMIUM	Gels.
GLONOINE	Glon.
GRAPHITES	Graph.
HEPAR SULPHURIS	Hep.s.
HYOSCYAMUS	Hyos.
HYPERICUM	Hyper.
IGNATIA	Ign.
IPECACUANHA	Ipec.
KALI BICHROMICUM	Kali.b.
KALI CARBONICUM	Kali.c.
KALI PHOSPHORICUM	Kali.p.
LAC CANINUM	Lac.c.
LACHESIS	Lach.
LEDUM	Led.
LYCOPODIUM	Lyc.
MAGNESIA PHOSPHORICA	Mag.p.
MERCURIUS SOLUBIS	Merc.s.
NATRUM CARBONICUM	Nat.c.
NATRUM MURIATICUM	Nat.m.
NATRUM SULPHURICUM	Nat.s.
NITRIC ACID	Nit.a.
NUX VOMICA	Nux.v.
OPIUM	Op.
PETROLEUM	Petr.
PHOSPHORIC ACID	Phos.ac.
PHOSPHORUS	Phos.
PHYTOLACCA	Phyt.
PLUMBUM	Plumb.
PODOPHYLLUM	Pod.
PULSATILLA	Puls.
RHUS TOXICODENDRON	Rhus t.
RUTA	Ruta.
SEPIA	Sep.
SILICA	Sil.
SPIGELIA	Spig.
SPONGIA	Spong.
STAPHISAGRIA	Staph.
STRAMONIUM	Stram.
SULPHUR	Sul.
THUJA	Thuj.
VERATRUM ALBUM	Ver.a.
ZINCUM METALLICUM	Zinc.

CHARACTERISTICS

ABDOMEN RETRACTED TO SPINE: Plumb.
ABDOMEN SUNKEN: Calc.p.
ABDOMINAL COMPLAINTS WORSE COFFEE: Canth.
ACHING: Phyt.
ACTIVITY GREAT, OF BODY: Coff.
ACTIVITY GREAT, OF MIND: Coff.
AFFECTIONATE: Phos.
AFFECTIONS PERIODICAL: China.
AFFECTIONS SPASMODIC: Cup.m.
AFFINITY FOR MUCOUS OUTLETS: Nit.a.
AGITATION: Cimic.
AILMENTS FROM VEXATION: Ipec.
AIR, DREADS OPEN: Calc.c.
AIR, MUST HAVE: Puls.
AIR, SENSITIVE TO COLD: Cocc.
AIR, SENSITIVE TO HOT: Cocc.
ALCOHOL INTOLERANCE: Sil.
ALONE BUT LIKES SOMEBODY IN HOUSE: Lyc.
ALONE DREADS TO BE: Sep.
ALONE FEARS TO BE: Stram.
ALONE WANTS TO BE WHEN CRYING: Nat.m.
ANAEMIA: Calc.p.
ANGER: Bell.; Nux v.; Puls.
ANGER SUPPRESSED: Staph.
ANGUISH: Ars.
ANKLES, WEAK: Nat.c.
ANTICIPATION: Lyc.
APATHY: Phos.ac.; Gels.
APPREHENSION: Arg.n.; Calc.c.; Caust.; Lyc.; Rhus t.
ANXIETY: Acon.; Arg.n.; Nux v.; Sep.; Sil.
ANXIETY FELT IN THE STOMACH: Kali c.
AVERSE TO FAT: Sep.
AVERSE TO MEAT: Sep.
AVERSE TO TOBACCO SMOKE: Ign.
AVERSE TO WORK: Sep.
AWKWARD, DROPS THINGS: Apis.

BAD-TEMPERED: Cham.
BACKACHE, WORSE MORNING BEFORE RISING: Staph.
BASHFUL: Bar.c.

BALL, SENSATION OF IN INNER PARTS: **Sep.**
BED, CANNOT REMAIN IN: **Rhus t.**
BILIOUS TEMPERAMENT: **Pod.**
BLACK EYE FROM BLOW: **Led.**
BLADDER IRRITABLE: **Staph.**
BLUE LINE ALONG MARGIN OF GUMS: **Plumb.**
BONE PAINS: **Aur.**
BREATHLESS: **Calc.c.**
BURNING: **Bell.; Phos.**

CAREFUL: **Nux v.**
CARTILAGE, ACTS ON: **Ruta.**
CHANGE, FEELS FROM DRY TO WET: **Nat.s.**
CHANGE, OF PAINS, IN CHARACTER: **Berb.**
CHANGE OF SYMPTOMS: **Berb.**
CHANGEABLE IN EVERYTHING: **Puls.**
CHILD CANNOT BEAR TO BE LOOKED AT: **Ant.c.**
CHILDISHNESS IN OLD PEOPLE: **Bar.c.**
CHILLY: **Bar.c.; Glon.**
CHILLY IN SPITE OF CLOTHING: **Nux v.**
CLAUSTROPHOBIC: **Arg.n.**
COLD BUT CRAVES FRESH AIR: **Graph.; Puls.**
COLD FEELS THE: **Sil.**
COLD WHATEVER COMPLAINT: **Led.**
COLDNESS: **Ver.a.**
COLDNESS ICY IN STOMACH: **Colch.**
COLLAPSE: **Ver.a.**
COMPLAINTS CAUSED OR ARE WORSE FROM WARM TO
COLD: **Dulc.**
COMPLAINTS AFTER BLEEDING: **China.**
COMPLAINTS AFTER DIARRHOEA: **China.**
COMPLAINTS AFTER EXCESSIVE LOSS OF FLUIDS: **China.**
COMPLAINTS DEVELOP SLOWLY: **Bry.**
COMPLAINTS FROM PENT UP WRATH: **Staph.**
COMPLAINTS FROM STRAINING FLEXOR TENDONS: **Ruta.**
CONGESTIONS, LOCAL, ESPECIALLY HEAD AND
CHEST: **Glon.**
CONSCIENTIOUS: **Puls.**
CONSOLATION, WORSE FROM: **Nat.m.**
CONSTIPATED, BETTER WHEN: **Calc.c.**
CONSTRICTION AS OF AN IRON BAND: **Cact.**
CONSTRICTION OF NECK AND WAIST: **Lach.**
CONTRADICTION, CANNOT BEAR: **Cocc.**

CONTRADICTIONS, FULL OF: Ign.
CONVULSIONS: Cup.m.; Zinc.
COSTIVE: Graph.
COUGH, CROUPY: Spong.
COUGH, LOOSE, WITH PAIN IN CHEST: Nat.s.
COUGH, WHEN ANY PART UNCOVERED: Hep.s.
COUGH, WHOOPING: Dros.
COUGH, WITH PAROXYSMS: Dros.
COWARDLY: Bar.c.
CRAMPS: Cup.m.; Mag.p.
CRAVES CHALK: Alum.
CRAVES CHARCOAL: Alum.
CRAVES COFFEE GROUNDS: Alum.
CRAVES EGGS: Calc.c.
CRAVES INDIGESTIBLE THINGS: Alum.; Calc.c.
CRAVES SALT: Nat.m.
CRAVES SOUR THINGS: Sep.
CRAVES SUGAR: Arg.n.
CRAVES SWEETS: Lyc.
CRAVES VINEGAR: Sep.
CROSS: Ant.c.
CRY, DESIRES TO: Amm.m.

DEBILITY: Ant.t.; China.; Nat.c.
DELIRIOUS, WILDLY: Stram.
DELUSIONS: Lac.c.
DEPRESSION: Phos.ac.; Caust.; Cimic.; Nat.m.; Nux v.; Pod.;
Sep.; Zinc.
DERANGEMENTS FROM OVER-LOADING STOMACH: Ant.c.
DESPAIR: Aur.
DIARRHOEA PRECEDED BY COLIC: Petr.
DIARRHOEA WORSE DAMP: Nat.s.
DISCHARGES BURNING: Ars.
DISCHARGES OFFENSIVE: Sul.
DISCHARGES TOUGH, STRINGY MUCUS: Kali b.
DISTENSION: Lyc.
DIZZINESS: Gels.
DREADS CROWDS: Arg.n.
DREADS MOTION, DOWNWARD: Bor.
DREAMS OF IMPENDING EVIL: Cimic.
DROWSINESS: Ant.t.; Gels.
DULLNESS: Gels.

EMACIATION RAPID: Plumb.; Thuj.
ERUPTIONS OOZING, HONEY-LIKE: Graph.
EXALTATION: Op.
EXCITED: Nux v.
EXHAUSTION: Ars.; Spong.
EXHAUSTION RAPID: Thuj.
EYE, SECRETIONS BLAND: All.c.

FACE FLUSHED: Bell.
FAINT: Calc.c.
FAINT WHEN HEAD IS RAISED: Bry.
FAINT WHEN KNEELING: Sep.
FAINT HEARTED: Sil.
FAIR: Calc.c.
FASTIDIOUS: Ars.; Nux v.
FAT: Calc.c.; Carb.v.; Graph.
FEAR: Acon.; Arg.n.; Ars.; Calc.c.; Gels.; Lac.c.
FEAR CAN VOMIT WITH: Acon.
FEAR COMPLAINTS FROM: Op.
FEAR OF BEING ALONE: Phos.
FEAR OF BEING TOUCHED: Kali c.
FEAR OF THE DARK: Phos.
FEAR OF DEATH: Acon.; Phos.
FEAR OF DISEASE: Phos.
FEAR OF FAILURE: Ars.
FEAR OF FUTURE: Acon.
FEAR OF SNAKES: Lac.c.
FEAR OF THUNDERSTORMS: Phos.
FEET AS THOUGH WEARING DAMP STOCKINGS: Calc.c.
FEET DAMP: Calc.c.
FEET FIDGETY: Zinc.
FEET WITH CORNS AND CALLOSITIES: Ant.c.
FEVERISH CONDITIONS AT NIGHT: Ant.c.
FINGERNAILS HORNY: Ant.c.
FINGERNAILS SPLIT: Ant.c.
FITFUL: Ant.c.
FLABBY: Calc.c.
FLATULENCE: Lyc.
FLOW THE GREATER, THE GREATER THE PAIN: Cimic.
FRIGHT: Ars.; Petr.
FRIGHT THE FEAR REMAINING: Op.
FRIGHTENED: Bor.
FULLNESS: Lyc.

FUNCTIONS SLUGGISH: **Alum.**
FUNKS EXAMINATIONS: **Arg.n.**

GLANDS ENLARGED: **Calc.c.**
GLOOM: **Aur.**
GRIEF: **Ign.**
GRIEF SILENT: **Puls.**
GRIT, WANT OF: **Sil.**
GROWS TOO FAST: **Phos.ac.**
GROWS TOO TALL: **Phos.ac.**

HAEMORRHAGE, BRIGHT: **Phos.**
HAEMORRHAGE, BRIGHT RED: **Ipec.**
HAEMORRHAGE, FREELY FLOWING: **Phos.**
HAEMORRHAGE, FROM ALL OUTLETS OF BODY: **Nit.a.**
HAEMORRHAGE, PROFUSE: **China.; Ipec.**
HAEMORRHAGE, WITH FAINTING: **China.**
HALLUCINATIONS: **Lac.c.**
HASTY: **Alum.**
HEAD, CANNOT BEAR ANYTHING ON: **Glon.**
HEAD, SYMPTOMS FROM INJURIES TO HEAD: **Nat.s.**
HEADACHE, BURSTING: **Glon.**
HEALING, PROMOTES HEALTHY: **Calen.**
HEART, VIOLENT BEATING: **Spig.**
HEAT, LACKS: **Led.**
HEAT, PARTICULARLY OF SKIN: **Phos.**
HEAVINESS AFTER SLIGHT EXERTION: **Spong.**
HEAVINESS FEELING OF, IN ALL ORGANS: **Amm.c.**
HEIGHTS, CANNOT LOOK DOWN FROM: **Arg.n.**
HUNGER, GNAWING: **Sep.**
HURRIED: **Alum.; Arg.n.**
HYPER SENSITIVITY, EXTREME NERVOUSNESS: **Amb.g.**
HYPER SENSITIVITY, TO ALL IMPRESSIONS: **Hep.s.**
HYSTERICAL: **Sep.**

IDEAS, FIXED: **Sil.**
ILL EFFECTS FROM ANGER: **Nat.m.**
ILL EFFECTS FROM FRIGHT: **Nat.m.**
ILL EFFECTS FROM GRIEF: **Nat.m.**
IMAGINATION, VIVID: **Op.**
IMPATIENT: **Cham.; Ipec.; Nit.a.; Nux v.**
IMPERFECT OXYDATION: **Carb.v.**
IMPULSES ON SEEING SHARP INSTRUMENTS: **Alum.**

IMPULSES ON SEEING BLOOD: Alum.
IMPULSIVE: Arg.n.
INDIFFERENCE: Phos.; Sep.
INJURIES TO NERVES: Hyper.
INTELLECTUALLY KEEN, PHYSICALLY WEAK: Lyc.
IRRATIONAL THOUGHTS: Arg.n.
IRRESOLUTE: Bar.c.
IRRESISTIBLE INCLINATION TO BITE TEETH OR GUMS
TOGETHER: Phyt.
IRRITABLE: Ant.t.; Bry.; Caust.; Cham.; Kali c.; Ipec.; Nat.m.:
Nux v.; Puls.; Sep.; Sil.
IRRITABILITY OF NERVOUS SYSTEM: Cocc.

JEALOUS, INSANELY: Apis.; Lach.
JERKY: Agar.
JUMPY: Sep.

LASSITUDE: Ant.t.
LAZY: Carb.v.; Sul.
LEARN, SLOW TO: Calc.p.
LIGHT, INTOLERANCE OF: Graph.
LOCKJAW, PREVENTS: Hyper.
LOQUACITY: Lach.; Pod.; Stram.

MAD IF IRRITATED: Ver.a.
MALICIOUS: Nux v.
MANIA: Hyos.; Ver.a.
MELANCHOLY: Cact.
MEMORY, LOSS OF: Anac.
MEMORY, WEAK: Bar.c.; Calc.p.
MENTAL EMOTIONS: Petr.
MENTAL STATES FOLLOWED BY LONG LASTING
COMPLAINTS: Petr.
MENTAL STRESS: Ign.
MIND, CONFUSION OF: Bapt.
MOODS CHANGEABLE: Ign.
MOODS VARIABLE: Alum.
MOODY: Nat.m.
MOTION, WORSE BY: Bry.
MOTOR PARALYSIS: Gels.
MOUTHFULS, FEW FILL UP: Lyc.
MOVEMENT, SLOWNESS IN: Calc.c.
MOVEMENT, QUICK: Nux v.

MOVES CONTINUALLY: **Phos.**
MUCOUS MEMBRANES DRY: **Alum.; Bry; Nat.m.**
MUCOUS MEMBRANES SECRETE PROFUSELY: **Dulc.**
MUCUS, GREAT ACCUMULATION, RATTLING: **Ant.t.**
MUSCULAR ATROPHY: **Plumb.**
MUSCULAR PROSTRATION: **Gels.**

NAILS THICK, MISS-SHAPEN: **Graph.**
NASAL DISCHARGE ACRID: **All.c.**
NAUSEA: **Ant.t.; Cup.m.**
NAUSEA PERSISTENT: **Ipec.**
NAUSEA UNRELIEVED BY VOMITING: **Ipec.**
NAUSEA AND VOMITING WITH CLEAN TONGUE: **Ipec.**
NERVE POWER, WANT OF: **Kali p.**
NERVOUS: **Sep.**
NERVOUS DREAD: **Kali p.**
NEURALGIAS: **Spig.**
NIGHT-WATCHING, EFFECTS OF: **Cocc.**
NUTRITION DEFECTIVE, UNABLE TO ASSIMILATE
CALCIUM: **Calc.p.**

OBESITY, TENDENCY TO: **Graph.**
OBSCENE: **Hyos.**
OFFENDED EASILY: **Nux v.; Sep.**
ONSET SUDDEN: **Acon.; Bell.**
ORIFICES RED: **Sul.**

PAINFULNESS, EXCESSIVE: **Hyper.**
PAINLESSNESS, ABNORMAL: **Op.**
PAINLESSNESS, OF MOST COMPLAINTS: **Stram.**
PAINS, AGONISING IN ABDOMEN, BENDS DOUBLE: **Colo.**
PAINS, BEARING DOWN, WORSE AFTER MENOPAUSE: **Agar.**
PAINS, BRUISED: **Arn.**
PAINS, BURNING: **Acon.; Apis.; Ars.; Canth.; Caust.**
PAINS, CONSTANT, UNDER INFERIOR ANGLE OF
SCAPULA: **Chel.**
PAINS, CONTRACTIVE: **Cup.m.**
PAINS, CUTTING: **Acon.; Kali c.**
PAINS, ERRATIC, ALTERNATING SIDES: **Lac.c.**
PAINS, NEURALGIC: **Mag.p.**
PAINS, NEURALGIC FOLLOWING AMPUTATION: **All.c.**
PAINS, NEURALGIC FOLLOWING INJURIES TO
NERVES: **All.c.**

PAINS, PINCHING: Phos.ac.

PAINS, PRICKING: Nit.a.

PAINS, PULSATING: Glon.

PAINS, RAW: Canth.; Caust.

PAINS, SEVERE FOLLOWING ABDOMINAL
OPERATION: Staph.

PAINS, SHARP: Agar.; Kali c.

PAINS, SMALL SPOTS, IN: Kali b.

PAINS, SORE: Arn.; Caust.

PAINS, SPASMODIC: Cact.

PAINS, SQUEEZING: Phos.ac.

PAINS, STABBING: Acon.

PAINS, STINGING: Acon.; Apis.

PAINS, STITCHING: Agar.; Bry.

PAINS, STOMACH, IN, WHEN EMPTY, BETTER
EATING: Anac.

PAINS, TEARING: Bry.

PAINS, TEARING IN UPPER HALF OF BRAIN: Amb.g.

PAINS, TRAVEL UPWARDS: Sep.

PAINS, VIOLENT: Cup.m.

PAINS, BETTER MOVEMENT: Bry.

PAINS, WORSE PRESSURE: Bry.

PALLOR: Ant.t.

PANTING: Cact.

PARALYSIS FROM EXPOSURE TO COLD, DRY WINDS: Caust.

PARALYSIS OF EXTENSOR MUSCLES: Plumb.

PARALYSIS OF SINGLE PARTS: Caust.

PARTICULAR: Nux v.

PARTS PAINFUL AS IF BRUISED: Ruta.

PEEVISH: Kali p.

PERIODICITY: Cact.

PERSPIRATION COLD: Ver.a.

PERSPIRATION PROFUSE, DOES NOT IMPROVE
CONDITION: Merc.s.

PHILOSOPHICAL: Sul.

PREVIOUS ILLNESS, NEVER RECOVERED FROM: Carb.v.

PROSTRATED: Ars.; Cact.; Colch.; Kali p.; Phyt.

PULSELESS: Cact.

PUNCTURE WOUNDS: Led.

PUPILS DILATED: Bell.

QUARRELSOME: Hyos.

QUIET, WANTS TO BE: Sep.

REDNESS: **Bell.**
RELATION SPECIFIC TO SKIN: **Dulc.**
RELATION SPECIFIC TO GLANDS: **Dulc.**
RESTLESSNESS, MENTAL: **Acon.**
RESTLESSNESS, PHYSICAL: **Acon.; Ars.; Cham.; Coff.; Phyt.;
Rhus t.**
RHEUMATISM INDUCED BY DAMP, COLD: **Dulc.**
RHEUMATISM TRAVELS UPWARDS FROM FEET: **Led.**
RHEUMATISM WORSE EVERY CHANGE TO COLD: **Dulc.**
RUBBED, DESIRES TO BE: **Phos.**

SADNESS: **Bar.c.; Cact.**
SADNESS PROFOUND: **Cocc.**
SALIVATION WITH INTENSE THIRST: **Merc.s.**
SAYS "NOTHING WRONG" WHEN VERY ILL: **Arn.**
SCORNFUL: **Ipec.**
SCRATCHING CHANGES LOCATION AND ITCHING: **Staph.**
SEASICKNESS: **Petr.**
SECRETIONS GLAIRY: **Amm.m.**
SECRETIONS PROFUSE: **Amm.m.**
SELFISH: **Sul.**
SENSATION AS IF CLAMPED WITH IRON BANDS: **Colo.**
SENSATION AS IF WIND BLOWING ON SOME PART: **Hep.s.**
SENSATION AS THOUGH PIERCED BY NEEDLE OF
ICE: **Agar.**
SENSATION OF COLDNESS BETWEEN
SHOULDERS: **Amm.m.**
SENSATION OF CONSTRICTION: **Apis.**
SENSATION OF EMPTINESS: **Cocc.**
SENSATION OF HOLLOWNESS: **Cocc.**
SENSITIVE: **Aur.; Coff.; Colch.; Phos.; Staph.**
SENSITIVE OVER: **Cham.; Ferr.m.**
SENSITIVE OVER TO LIGHT: **Nux v.**
SENSITIVE OVER TO MUSIC: **Nux v.**
SENSITIVE OVER TO NOISE: **Nux v.**
SENSITIVE OVER TO ODOUR: **Nux v.**
SENSITIVE TO ALL IMPRESSIONS: **Sil.**
SENSITIVE TO COLD: **Calc.c.**
SENSITIVE TO COLD, DAMP: **Calc.c.**
SENSITIVE TO HEAT AND COLD: **Merc.s.**
SENSITIVE TO SUDDEN NOISE: **Bor.**
SENSITIVE TO SUN: **Calc.c.**
SENSITIVE TO TOUCH: **Spig.**

SELF-WILLED: Sil.

SEPTIC CONDITIONS: Bapt.

SICK IF EATS RICH, FAT FOOD: Puls.

SIDES – LEFT: Lach.

SIDES – RIGHT AND MOVES LEFT: Lyc.

SIDES – ONE PARALYZED THE OTHER CONVULSED: Stram.

SIGHING: Ign.

SINKING FEELING, MORNING: Sul.

SKIN BURNING: Bell.; Sul.

SKIN DIRTY: Caust.

SKIN DRY: Bell.

SKIN ERUPTIONS WORSE WINTER, BETTER SUMMER: Petr.

SKIN HOT: Bell.

SKIN ITCHING: Sul.

SKIN PALLOR OF: Ferr.m.

SKIN PERSPIRING: Apis.

SKIN SALLOW: Caust.

SKIN WHITE: Caust.

SLEEP – CATNAP: Sul.

SLEEP RESTLESS: Bell.

SLEEP WAKENS FROM, WITH SENSE OF
SUFFOCATION: Spong.

SLEEPINESS: Ant.t.

SLEEPLESSNESS: Ant.t.

SLEEPS INTO AGGRAVATION: Lach.

SLEEPY, BUT CANNOT: Op.

SLUGGISH: Carb.v.

SMELL OF COOKING BRINGS FAINTNESS AND
NAUSEA: Colch.

SNAPPISH: Cham.

SOBBING: Ign.

SORENESS: Phyt.

SORENESS GREAT MUSCULAR: Bapt.

SOURNESS OF STOOL: Calc.c.

SOURNESS OF SWEAT: Calc.c.

SOURNESS OF TASTE: Calc.c.

SOURNESS OF URINE: Calc.c.

SPITEFUL: Phyt.

STANDING, WORSE: Sul.

STITCHES IN ANY PART OF BODY: Kali c.

STRANGERS, DREAD OF: Bar.c.

SUDDENNESS OF ATTACKS: Bapt.

SUDDENNESS OF RECOVERY: Bapt.

SUICIDE, WANTS TO COMMIT: **Aur.**
SULLEN: **Nux v.**
SUNSTROKE: **Glon.**
SUNSTROKE CHRONIC EFFECTS OF: **Nat.c.**
SUPPURATIONS: **Sil.**
SUPPURATIONS TENDENCY TO: **Hep.s.**
SURGING OF BLOOD FROM HEAD TO HEART: **Glon.**
SUSPECTS EVERYONE AROUND HIM: **Anac.**
SUSPICIOUS: **Apis.**
SWEAT COLD: **Calc.c.**
SWEAT ONLY ON COVERED PARTS: **Thuj.**
SWEAT PROFUSE: **Calc.c.**
SWEATS: **Ant.t.**
SWEATS ESPECIALLY ON HEAD: **Calc.c.**
SWEATS IN COLD ROOM: **Calc.c.**
SWEATS WITHOUT THIRST: **Apis.**
SYMPATHETIC, INTENSELY: **Caust.**
SYMPATHY, HATES: **Sep.**
SYMPATHY, LOVES: **Puls.**
SYMPTOMS APPEAR DIAGONALLY: **Agar.**
SYMPTOMS CAUSED BY EXPOSURE TO COLD, DRY
WINDS: **Acon.**
SYMPTOMS SPASMODIC: **Mag.p.**
SYMPTOMS WORSE LIGHT: **Merc.s.**
SYMPTOMS WORSE SEA AIR: **Nat.m.**

TALK AMOROUS: **Ver.a.**
TALK LASCIVIOUS: **Ver.a.**
TALK LEWD: **Ver.a.**
TALK RELIGIOUS: **Ver.a.**
TALKS TO IMAGINARY PEOPLE: **Hyos.**
TEA, ANTIDOTE TO: **Thuj.**
TEARFUL: **Apis.**
TEARS FREQUENT: **Puls.**
TEMPER, CANNOT CONTROL: **Cham.**
TEMPERAMENT FIERY: **Nux v.**
TEMPERAMENT GENTLE: **Puls.**
TEMPERAMENT MILD: **Puls.**
TEMPERATURE, SUDDEN RISE IN: **Bell.**
TENSION: **Acon.**
THINKING, SLOWNESS OF: **Cocc.**
THIRST: **Ars.; Nat.m.**
THIRST EXCESSIVE: **Bry.**

THIRST FOR COLD DRINKS, VOMITED AS SOON AS
WARM: Phos.
THIRST LACK OF: Ant.t.
THIRSTLESS: Apis.; Puls.
TIME PASSES TOO QUICKLY: Cocc.
TIMID: Bar.c.; Caust.
TIREDNESS: Gels.
TONGUE FLABBY: Merc.s.
TONGUE LARGE: Merc.s.
TONGUE THICKLY COATED WHITE: Ant.c.
TONGUE TRIANGULAR TIP RED: Rhus t.
TRAUMATIC INJURIES, AFTER: Arn.
TREMBLING: Agar.; Merc.s.; Phos.; Zinc.
TWITCHING: Agar.; Hyos.; Ign.
TWITCHING OF SINGLE MUSCLE: Zinc.

ULCERS, PRICKING: Nit.a.
UNDER NOURISHED: Sil.
UNHAPPINESS: Ign.
UNCONSCIOUS: Phos.ac.
UNCOVER, DESIRES TO: Hyos.
UNTIDY: Sul.
UPPER PART OF BODY THIN, LOWER DROPSICAL: Lyc.
URINATE, CONSTANT, INTOLERABLE URGE: Canth.
URINE, STRONG SMELLING – LIKE HORSE'S: Nit.a.

VACCINATION, ILL EFFECTS OF: Thuj.
VEXATIONS: Petr.
VIOLENT ATTACKS: Bell.
VOMITING: Ant.t.
VOMITING PROFUSE: Ver.a.
VOMITING VIOLENT: Ver.a.

WANTS LIGHT AND COMPANY: Stram.
WATER, DISLIKE OF: Sul.
WEAK, EMPTY SENSATION IN STOMACH NOT BETTER
EATING: Ign.
WEAKENED BY AGE: Amb.g.
WEAKENED BY OVERWORK: Amb.g.
WEAKNESS: Ant.t.; Hyos.; Merc.s.; Nat.m.
WEAKNESS FROM SPEAKING OR WALKING ALTHOUGH
LOOKS STRONG: Ferr.m.
WEAKNESS MENTAL: Bar.c.; Phos.ac.

WEAKNESS PHYSICAL: **Bar.c.; Phos.ac.; Phos.**
WEATHER, COLD CANNOT BE TOLERATED: **Kali c.**
WEATHER, WORSE IN HOT: **Pod.**
WEEPS WHEN TELLING SYMPTOMS: **Sep.**
WEEPS WHEN THANKED: **Lyc.**
WHINING: **Apis.**
WIND EXCESSIVE IN LOWER ABDOMEN: **Lyc.**
WORRY: **Ars.**
WOUNDS, PUNCTURED: **Hyper.**
WRIST-DROP: **Plumb.**

YELLOW EYES: **Chel.**
YELLOW FACE: **Chel.**
YELLOW SKIN: **Chel.**
YELLOW URINE: **Chel.**
YIELDING: **Sil.**

MIND

ABSENT MINDED: Arn.; Lac.c.
ACTIVITY UNUSUAL: Coff.
ADAPTED TO DISAPPOINTED LOVE: Coff.
ADAPTED TO LAUGHTER, EXCESSIVE: Coff.
ADAPTED TO MENTAL SHOCK: Coff.
ADAPTED TO MOODS: Coff.
AILMENTS FROM ANGER: Lyc.; Op.
AILMENTS FROM CHAGRIN: Phos.ac.
AILMENTS FROM FRIGHT: Lyc.; Op.
AILMENTS FROM GRIEF: Phos.ac.
AILMENTS FROM HOMESICKNESS: Phos.ac.
AILMENTS FROM JOY, EXCESSIVE: Op.
AILMENTS FROM LOVE, DISAPPOINTED: Phos.ac
AILMENTS FROM MORTIFICATION: Lyc.
AILMENTS FROM SHAME: Op.
AILMENTS FROM SORROW: Phos.ac.
AILMENTS FROM TERROR: Op.
AILMENTS FROM VEXATION: Lyc.
ALONE, DISLIKES BEING: Lyc., Phos.
ALONE, DOESN'T WANT TO TALK: Colo.
ANGER: Colo.; Staph.
ANGER FROM LEAST CONTRADICTION: Aur.
ANGERED EASILY: Lyc.
ANXIETY: Ant.t.; Bor.; Dros.; Graph.; Nat.c.; Nit.a.; Phos., Spong.; Stram.; Sul.
ANXIETY IN STOMACH: Kali c.
APATHETIC: Gels.; Phos.ac.; Phos.; Sep.; Thuj.
APPREHENSION: Arg.n.; Calc.c.; Graph.; Lyc.; Rhus t.
ATTENTION, DIFFICULTY IN FIXING: Sil.

BASHFUL: Bar.c.
BRAIN FAG: Anac.; Kali p.

CHANGE, WANTS CONSTANT: Hep.s.
CHILDISHNESS IN OLD PEOPLE: Bar.c.
CHILDREN CANNOT BEAR TO BE TOUCHED: Ant.t.
CLAUSTROPHOBIA: Arg.n.
COMPLAINTS, FEELS MORE WHEN THINKING ABOUT THEM: Calc.p.
COMPLAINTS, FROM ANGER: Bry.

COMPLAINTS, FROM FRIGHT: Bry.
COMPLAINTS, FROM RESENTMENT: Bry.
CONCENTRATING, WORSE WHEN: Nat.c.
CONFIDENCE, LOSS OF: Anac.
CONFUSED: Bar.c.; Glon.; Thuj.
CONFUSED AS TO TIME: Lach.
CONSCIOUSNESS, LOSS OF: Op.
CONSOLATION AGGRAVATES: Nat.m.
CONVULSIONS: Cup.m.
COWARDLY: Bar.c.
CRAVES COMPANY: Phos.
CRYING THEN LAUGHING: Coff.
CURSE, DESIRES TO: Anac.

DAZED: Thuj.
DEATH, THINKS IT'S NEAR: Petr.
DEATH, THINKS OF NOTHING BUT: Graph.
DEBILITY FROM SUMMER HEAT: Nat.c.
DEBILITY NERVOUS: Zinc.
DECISIONS, UNABLE TO MAKE: Graph.
DEJECTED, FEELS: Aur.; Dros.
DELIRIUM: Petr.
DELIRIUM AT NIGHT: Lach.
DELIRIUM NOISY, WITH HALLUCINATIONS: Stram.
DELUSIONS: Lac.c.; Plumb.
DELUSIONS OF IMPENDING MISFORTUNE: Ver.a.
DEPRESSED: Anac.; Cimic.; Hep.s.; Lach.; Nat.c.; Nat.m.; Nat.s.;
Nit.a.; Petr.; Plumb.; Pod.
DESIRE TO GET WELL: Sep.
DESIRES COMPANY: Apis.
DESPAIR: Nit.a.; Ruta.
DESPONDENT: Graph.; Puls.
DIFFICULT TO GET ON WITH: Hep.s.
DISCONTENTED: Led.
DISGUST OF LIFE: Aur.
DISHEARTENED: Dros.
DISTURBED, DOES NOT WANT TO BE: Bry.
DREAD OF MEN: Lyc.
DREAMS OF IMPENDING EVIL: Cimic.
DULLNESS: Gels.; Staph.
DWARFISH GROWTH OF YOUNG PEOPLE: Bar.c.

EMOTION CAN CAUSE FAINTING: Cham.

EMOTIONAL: **Coff.; Op.**
EMOTIONAL INSTABILITY: **Apis.**
EMOTIONAL STRESS CAUSES PHYSICAL SYMPTOMS: **Ars.**
ESCAPE, DESIRES TO: **Bell.**
EXASPERATION, TOSSING ABOUT IN ANGUISH: **Coff.**
EXASPERATION, WITH TEARS: **Coff.**
EXCITABLE: **Nit.a.**
EXCITEMENT: **Sil.; Stram.**
EXHAUSTED WHEN ILL: **Colch.**

FEAR, INTANGIBLE: **Acon.**
FEAR OF BED: **Acon.**
FEAR OF BEING TOUCHED: **Arn.**
FEAR OF THE DARK: **Acon.**
FEAR OF DEATH: **Acon.; Cact.; Lac.c.**
FEAR OF DISEASE: **Lac.c.**
FEAR OF DOWNWARD MOTION: **Bor.**
FEAR OF FALLING: **Lac.c.**
FEAR OF GHOSTS: **Acon.**
FEAR OF LOSS OF REASON: **Calc.c.**
FEAR OF MISFORTUNE: **Calc.c.**
FEAR OF POVERTY: **Bry.**
FEAR OF SHARP, POINTED THINGS: **Spig.**
FEAR OF SNAKES: **Lac.c.**
FEAR OF THUNDER: **Phos.**
FEAR WITH DIFFICULT BREATHING: **Spong.**
FEAR, VOMITS WITH: **Acon.**
FEARFUL: **Apis.; Arg.n.; Bell.; Bry.; Stram.**
FIDGETY: **Bor.**
FOOLISH: **Hyos.**
FORGETFUL: **Arn.; Calc.c.; Lac.c.; Merc.s.; Petr.**
FRIGHT, SPASMS OF: **Op.**
FRIGHTENED: **Kali c.**
FRUSTRATION: **Sep.**
FURIOUS OVER PETTY THINGS: **Hep.s.**
FURY: **Bell.**
FUTURE, CONCERNED ABOUT: **Dros.**

GRIEF, FULL OF: **Aur.**

HALLUCINATIONS: **Plumb.**
HALLUCINATIONS IN DAYLIGHT: **Lac.c.**
HURRIED: **Arg.n.; Nat.m.**

HURRIED TALKING: Merc.s.

IDEAS FIXED: Thuj.
IDEAS FULL OF: Coff.
ILLUSIONS, FANTASTIC: Bell.
IMAGINATIONS, FULL OF STRANGE: Phos.
IMPETUOUS: Hep.s.
IMPULSIVE: Hep.s.
INDIFFERENT: Apis.; Nat.m.; Phos.ac.; Phos.; Sep.; Staph.; Sul.; Ver.a.
INDISPOSED TO EVERYTHING: Sul.
INDOLENCE OF MIND: Sul.
INTELLECTUAL SUFFERING: Lyc.
IRRATIONAL: Stram.
IRRESOLUTE: Anac.; Bar.c.; Lac.c.; Puls.
IRRITABILITY: Ant.t.; Bry.; Colo.; Hep.s.; Nat.s.; Nit.a.; Petr.; Sep.
IRRITABILITY EXCESSIVE: Ant.t.; Apis.

JOYLESS: Apis.

LANGOUR: Gels.
LASSITUDE: Sul.
LAUGHTER, EXCESSIVE: Coff.
LETHARGIC: Zinc.
LISTLESS: Gels.
LOCATION, LOSS OF: Glon.
LOQUACITY: Agar.; Pod.
LOVE, DISAPPOINTED: Coff.

MANIA, ACUTE: Canth.
MELANCHOLY: Lyc.; Sul.
MELANCHOLY FROM ANGER: Cham.
MEMORY DEFICIENT, FORGETS IN THE MIDDLE: Bar.c.
MEMORY LOSS OF: Anac.; Bar.c.
MEMORY POOR: Hep.s.; Lach.; Merc.s.
MEMORY WEAK: Anac.; Nit.a.
MENTAL ACTIVITY CAUSES SLEEPLESSNESS: Coff.
MENTAL CONFUSION: Dulc.
MENTAL EXERTION, WORSE FROM: Kali p.
MENTAL AND PHYSICAL EXHAUSTION FROM OVER-EXERTION OF MIND: Cup.m.
MENTAL AND PHYSICAL EXHAUSTION FROM LOSS OF SLEEP: Cup.m.

MENTAL WEAKNESS: Bar.c.
MIND CALMNESS CONTRA INDICATES: Cham.
MIND DISTURBED: Nat.s.
MIND IN AN UPROAR: Stram.
MIND WEAK: Bar.c.
MISERABLE: Petr.
MISTRUSTS: Dros.; Merc.s.
MOODS CHANGEABLE: Ign.

NERVE STRAIN: Phos.ac.
NERVES WEAKENED, WITH GREAT DEBILITY: Kali c.
NERVOUS: Bor.; Nit.a.; Nux v.
NERVOUS HYPERSENSITIVITY: Amb.g.
NERVOUS SYSTEM, ACTS ON: Coff.
NERVOUS WORN OUT: Amb.g.
NIGHT TERRORS: Kali p.
NOISE, SLIGHT, UNBEARABLE: Ferr.m.
NUMBNESS: Phos.

PAIN AS IF BALL ROSE FROM THROAT TO BRAIN: Plumb.
PASSION, VIOLENT OUTBURSTS: Staph.
PEEVISH: Amm.m.; Dros.; Thuj.
PERCEPTION SLOW: Plumb.
PRIDE: Sul.
PROSTRATION: Kali p.; Phos.

QUARRELSOME: Hep.s.; Nux v.; Petr.

RAGE: Stram.
REPROACHES OTHERS: Nux v.
RESTLESS: Ant.t.; Arg.n.; Graph.; Nat.c.; Rhus t.; Sep.
RESTLESS CHANGES FROM ONE THING TO
ANOTHER: Dros.
RESTLESS INTERNAL: Sil.

SAD: Apis.; Bar.c.; Cocc.; Graph.; Hep.s.; Lach.; Nat.m.; Nux v.;
Rhus t.
SELF PITY: Graph.
SENILE DEMENTIA: Bar.c.
SENSATION OF ACUTE INTOLERABLE PAIN: Colch.
SENSATION OF OPENING AND SHUTTING OF BRAIN: Cimic.
SENSE OF UNREALITY: Lac.c.
SENSES MORE ACUTE: Coff.

SENSITIVE: Bor.; Kali c.
SENSITIVE HYPER: Phos.
SENSITIVE OVER, TO PAIN: Lyc.
SENSITIVE TO NOISE: Aur.; Nat.c.; Nit.a.; Zinc.
SENSITIVE TO WHAT IS SAID ABOUT HER: Staph.
SENSITIVENESS, EMOTIONAL: Thuj.
SENSITIVITY, EXTREME: Nux v.; Thuj.
SHOCK FROM INJURIES, REMOVES: Arn.
SIGHING: Ign.
SLUGGISHNESS: Phos.
SOBBING: Ign.
SOLITUDE, DREADS: Sep.
STRANGERS, DREAD OF: Bar.c.
STUPIDITY: Stram.; Zinc.
STUPOR, DEEP: Hyos.
SUDDENNESS OF SYMPTOMS: Bell.
SUICIDE, TALKS OF COMMITTING: Aur.
SUICIDE, TENDENCY TO: Nat.s.
SULLEN: Ver.a.
SURPRISES, SUDDEN: Coff.
SUSPICIOUS: Anac.; Hyos.
SWEAR, DESIRES TO: Anac.
SYMPTOMS, EMOTIONAL FROM WEAKNESS: China.
SYMPTOMS, MENTAL FROM TIREDNESS AND
WEAKNESS: China.
SYMPTOMS, FROM FEAR: Sep.
SYMPTOMS, FROM STRAIN: Sep.

TALKING, RAPID: Merc.s.
THINKING BRINGS ON HEADACHE: Nat.c.
THINKING DIFFICULT: Sil.
THOUGHTS, CANNOT COLLECT: Phos.ac.
TIMID: Bar.c.; Puls.
TIREDNESS: Phos.ac.
TRAUMA, REMOVES: Arn.
TREMBLING: Phos.
TURMOIL IN BRAIN: Bell.

UNEASINESS, EXCESSIVE: Nux v.

VIOLENCE: Stram.

WEAKNESS: Arn.; Ruta.; Sil

WEAKNESS MENTAL AND BODILY: **Bar.c.**
WEARINESS: **Arn.; Sil.**
WEEPING CAUSED BY MUSIC: **Graph.**
WEEPING INVOLUNTARY: **Nat.m.**
WEEPS ALL DAY :   **Lyc.**
WEEPS EASILY: **Puls.**
WEEPS WITHOUT KNOWING WHY: **Rhus t.**
WILLS, FEELS AS THOUGH HE HAS TWO: **Anac.**

HEAD

BAND FEELING ROUND HEAD: Gels.; Merc.s.; Nit.a.
BLOOD, RUSH OF, TO HEAD ON WAKING: Lyc.
BRAIN, BASE OF, HOT: Zinc.
BRAIN, CONCUSSION: Hyper.
BRAIN, FEELS LOOSE: Nat.s.
BURNING IN VERTEX: Graph.
BUZZING: Phos.ac.

COLDNESS, ICY RIGHT SIDE: Calc.c.
COLDNESS FROM NAPE OF NECK OVER HEAD, WHICH
FEELS HEAVY: Chel.
CONFUSION: Phos.ac.
COVERED, CANNOT BEAR TO BE: Glon.

DANDRUFF: Nat.m.
DISPROPORTIONATELY LARGE FOR BODY: Bar.c.
DIZZINESS FROM SUNLIGHT: Agar.
DIZZINESS SENILE: Amb.g.
DRUNKEN CONFUSION: Nux v.
DRUNKEN GIDDINESS: Nux v.
DULL: Nat.m.

ELONGATED, FEELS: Hyper.
ERUPTION MOIST ON SCALP: Petr.

FEELS HEAVY: Bapt.
FEELS NUMB: Bapt.
FEELS TOO LARGE: Bapt.
FOREHEAD, COLD SWEAT ON: Ver.a.

HAIR FALLS OUT EASILY: Carb.v.
HEADACHE, ALTERNATING WITH DIARRHOEA: Pod.
HEADACHE, BACK OF HEAD: Spig.
HEADACHE, BATHING, AFTER: Ant.c.
HEADACHE, BURSTING: Glon.; Merc.s.; Nat.m.
HEADACHE, CATARRHAL: Merc.s.
HEADACHE, CONGESTIVE: Cact.; Ferr.m.; Ign.
HEADACHE, EXPOSED TO SUN, WHEN: Lach.
HEADACHE, FRONTAL: All.c.; Arg.n.

HEADACHE, INTENSE: **Phyt.**

HEADACHE, MORNING: **Agar.; Sep.**

HEADACHE, NERVOUS: **Thuj.**

HEADACHE, NEURALGIC, EXCRUCIATING: **Mag.p.**

HEADACHE, OCCIPITAL: **Gels.; Nux v.; Petr.; Phos.ac.**

HEADACHE, OVER EYEBROWS: **Kali b.**

HEADACHE, OVER LEFT EYE: **Spig.**

HEADACHE, PULSATING: **Ferr.m.; Glon.**

HEADACHE, RHEUMATIC, EXCRUCIATING: **Mag.p.**

HEADACHE, SICK, WITH NAUSEA: **Ipec.**

HEADACHE, SLEEPS INTO: **Lach.**

HEADACHE, SYCOTIC: **Thuj.**

HEADACHE, SYPHILITIC: **Thuj.**

HEADACHE, THROBBING, INTENSE: **China.**

HEADACHE, FROM ANY OVER INDULGENCE: **Carb.v.**

HEADACHE, FROM COLD WIND: **Kali c.**

HEADACHE, FROM DISORDERED STOMACH: **Ant.c.**

HEADACHE, FROM MENTAL EXERTION: **Coff.**

HEADACHE, FROM OVERWORK: **Puls.**

HEADACHE, FROM TALKING: **Coff.**

HEADACHE, FROM THINKING: **Coff.**

HEADACHE, ONE SIDED: **Coff.; Spig.**

HEADACHE, WITH AVERSION TO MANY FOODS: **Sep.**

HEADACHE, WITH COLDNESS: **Arg.n.**

HEADACHE, WITH FEELING OF EMPTY STOMACH: **Sep.**

HEADACHE, WITH NAUSEA: **Sep.**

HEADACHE, WITH NOSEBLEED: **Sep.**

HEADACHE, WITH SOUR VOMITING: **Nux v.**

HEADACHE, WITH STUPIFYING PAIN: **Staph.**

HEADACHE, WITH VERTIGO: **Sep.**

HEADACHE, WORSE EATING: **Nux v.**

HEADACHE, BETTER UNCOVERING: **Lyc.**

HEAT, CANNOT BEAR ON: **Glon.**

HEAT, ON TOP OF HEAD: **Nat.s; Sul.**

HEAVINESS: **Puls.**

HEAVY: **Ign.; Nat.m.; Petr.**

HOLLOW: **Ign.**

HOT: **Arn.**

HOT VERY: **Stram.**

INTOXICATION: **Nux v.**

JERKS HEAD FREQUENTLY FROM PILLOW: **Stram.**

LIGHTNESS OF HEAD IN OLD PEOPLE: Op.

NEURALGIA: Thuj.

PAIN, ACHING: Gels.
PAIN, AS IF FROM A FALL: Ruta.
PAIN, BACK OF HEAD: Zinc.
PAIN, BACK OF HEAD AFTER INJURY TO HEAD: Nat.s.
PAIN, BORING, BETTER PRESSURE: Arg.n.
PAIN, IN TEMPLES: Gels.; Lyc.
PAIN, NAPE OF NECK: Phos.ac.
PAIN, NEURALGIC: Puls.
PAIN, PRESSING: Nat.m.; Nat.s.
PAIN, SHOOTING: Ruta.
PAIN, TEARING: Phos.ac.
PAIN, VIOLENT, ESPECIALLY AT NIGHT: Aur.
PAIN, WITH FEELING OF FULLNESS: Bell.
PAINFUL TO TOUCH: Merc.s.
PRESSURE: Phos.ac.
PRESSURE IN FOREHEAD: Nat.s.; Phyt.
PRESSURE ON: Lach.

ROLLING FROM SIDE TO SIDE: Pod.

SCALDHEAD WITH THICK BROWN CRUSTS: Dulc.
SCALP, BONES OF, SORE: Kali b.
SCALP, DRY: Sul.
SCALP ITCHING: Sul.
SCALP WOUNDS, HEALS: Calen.
SENSATION OF BEING TOUCHED BY ICY COLD
HAND: Hyper.
SENSATION OF BURSTING: Acon.; Sil.
SENSATION OF HEAT: Acon.
SENSATION OF HEAVINESS: Acon.
SENSATION OF LUMP OF ICE ON VERTEX: Ver.a.
SENSATION OF SQUEEZING: Phos.ac.
SENSATION OF SURGING: Sep.
SENSATION OF SURGING FROM HEAD TO HEART: Glon.
SENSATION OF TIGHT CAP OVER SCALP: Berb.
SENSATION OF UNDULATING, AS MOVING IN WAVES: Glon.
SENSATION OF WEIGHT ON TOP: Zinc.
SENSATION OF WEIGHT ON VERTEX: Cact.
SENSITIVE TO COLD ABOUT: Bar.c.

SHOCKS THROUGH HEAD, EYES, EARS WHEN PRESSING
TEETH TOGETHER: **Amm.c.**
SWEAT, PROFUSE ON: **Sil.**
SWEATING, WETS PILLOW: **Calc.c.**

VERTIGO: **Gels.**
VERTIGO, GIDDY ON RISING: **Rhus t.**
VERTIGO ON RISING: **Petr.; Phos.; Nit.ac.**
VERTIGO WHEN TURNING HEAD TO LEFT: **Colo.**
VERTIGO WITH NAUSEA, ESPECIALLY WHEN RIDING OR
SITTING UP: **Cocc.**
VERTIGO WORSE SITTING: **Puls.**

WORSE STOOPING: **Ign.**
WORSE WRAPPING UP HEAD: **Sil.**

EYES

ACHING: Merc.s.
ACHING IN AND OVER: Ruta.
BLOATING ROUND EYES: Phos.
BURNING: All.c.; Alum.; Bell.; Puls.

CANTHI FISSURED: Ant.c.
CANTHI RAW: Ant.c.
COLD SETTLES IN EYES WITH THICK YELLOW
DISCHARGE: Dulc.
CONJUNCTIVITIS CHRONIC: Nat.s.
CORNEA, SPOTS ON: Calc.c.
CORNEA, ULCERS ON: Calc.c.

DAZZLED BY FIRELIGHT: Merc.s.
DISCHARGE ACRID: Merc.s.
DISCHARGE BLAND: Puls.
DISCHARGE PROFUSE: Puls.
DISCHARGE ROPY: Kali b.
DISCHARGE STRINGY: Kali b.
DISCHARGE THICK: Puls.
DISCHARGE THIN: Merc.s.
DISCHARGE TOUGH: Kali b.
DISCHARGE YELLOW: Kali b.; Puls.
DOUBLE VISION: Agar.
DRY: Acon.; Alum.; Bell.

EYE-BALLS HURT: Calc.p.
EYE-BALLS INTENSE ITCHING: Cimic.
EYE-LASHES STICK TOGETHER: Bor.
EYE-LIDS AGGLUTINATED: Puls.; Rhus t.
EYE-LIDS BURNING: Sul.
EYE-LIDS CLOSE INVOLUNTARILY: Sep.
EYE-LIDS COVERED WITH SCABS: Petr.
EYE-LIDS ECZEMA OF: Graph.
EYE-LIDS HEAVY: Gels.; Rhus t.
EYE-LIDS INFLAMED: Petr.; Puls.
EYE-LIDS RED: Acon.; Graph.; Lyc.; Petr.; Rhus t
EYE-LIDS STIFF: Rhus t.
EYE-LIDS SWOLLEN: Acon.; Graph.; Rhus t.
EYE-LIDS ULCERATION OF: Sul.

FIERY LOOK: Canth.

HOT: Acon.

INFLAMMATION: Rhus t.
INFLAMMATION OF WHITE OF EYE: Staph.
ITCHING: Puls.
ITCHING EYE-BALLS: Merc.s.
ITCHING LOWER LIDS: Ruta.

LACHRYMATION BLAND. WITH A COLD: All.c.
LACHRYMATION BURNING :   Merc.s.
LACHRYMATION EXCORIATING: Merc.s.
LACHRYMATION HOT: Apis
LACHRYMATION PROFUSE: Merc.s.; Phyt.
LACHRYMATION SMARTING: All.c.
LIGHT, WANTS: Stram.

MISTY: Merc.s.
MUSCLES STIFF: Nat.m.
MUSCLES TWITCHING: Agar.; Gels.
MUSCLES WEAK: Nat.m.

NEURALGIA, ORBITAL: Gels.
NIGHT-BLINDNESS: Lyc.

OPENING EYES DIFFICULT: Rhus t.
OPTIC NERVE INFLAMED: Plumb.

PAIN BORING, BETTER PRESSURE: Colo.
PAIN EXTENDING TO SOCKETS: Spig.
PAIN PRESSING: Phos.ac.
PAIN PRESSING ON TURNING EYES: Spig.
PAIN SEVERE IN AND AROUND: Spig.
PAIN SHARP: Nit.a.
PAIN SHARP BETTER PRESSURE: Colo.
PAIN STICKING: Nit.a.
PHOTOPHOBIA: Aur.; Phos.
PRESSURE, FEELING OF: China.; Nat.m.; Petr.
PUFFY, BAGS UNDER: Apis.
PUPILS DILATED: Bell.; Hyos.; Stram.
PUPILS DILATION CHRONIC: Calc.c.

ROLLING: Zinc.

SCURFY MARGIN OF LIDS: Staph.
SENSATION OF BLUNT OBJECT PUSHED IN: Ruta.
SENSATION OF FIRE IN: Ruta.
SENSATION OF HEAT IN: Ruta.
SENSATION OF SAND IN: Sep.
SENSITIVE TO LIGHT: All.c.
SIGHT DIM: Gels.; Merc.s.
SIGHT WEAKNESS OF: Ign.
SMALL OBJECTS LOOK LARGE: Stram.
SMARTING: Alum.; Nit.a.; Phyt.
SMARTING IN RIGHT EYE: Sep.
SPASM, LOWER LID: Ruta.
SQUINTING: Zinc.
STARING: Bell.; Canth.; Hyos.; Stram.
STYES: Lyc.; Puls.; Staph.
SWELLING OVER UPPER EYELIDS: Kali c.
SWOLLEN, FEEL: Bell.

TIRED: Ruta.

ULCERATION: OF EYE-LIDS: Lyc.
ULCERS ON CORNEA: Hep.s.

VISION BLURRED: Ruta.
VISION WEAK: Nat.m.; Ruta.

WHITES OF EYES VERY YELLOW: Plumb.

EARS

BURNING: **Agar.**
BUZZING IN: **Kali p.**

CARTILAGE AND UNDER MASTOID PROCESS, PAINS AS IF
FROM BELOW OR FALL: **Ruta.**
CRACKING IN: **Petr.**
CRACKING IN WHEN CHEWING: **Nit.a.**

DEAFNESS: **Hyos.; Nit.a.**
DEAFNESS ESPECIALLY TO HUMAN VOICE: **Phos.**
DEAFNESS IN DAMP WEATHER: **Calen.**
DRYNESS OF INNER EARS: **Graph.**

ECZEMA: **Lyc.**
ERUPTION BEHIND: **Graph.**

FEEL AS IF FROZEN: **Agar.**

GLANDS ENLARGED: **Calc.c.**
GLANDS PAINFUL: **Bar.c.**
GLANDS SWOLLEN: **Bar.c.**

HEARING BETTER IN NOISE: **Graph.**
HEARING HARDNESS OF: **Bar.c.; Lyc.**
HEARING IMPAIRED: **Amb.g.**
HEARING REDUCED: **Petr.**
HUMMING IN: **Kali p.; Lyc.**

INFLAMMATION, EXTERNAL: **Merc.s.**
INFLAMMATION, INTERNAL: **Merc.s.**
ITCHING: **Agar.**

MOISTURE, BEHIND: **Graph.**
MUCUS FOETID: **Kali b.**
MUCUS STRINGY: **Kali b.**
MUCUS TOUGH: **Kali b.**
MUCUS YELLOW: **Kali b.**
NEURALGIC PAINS: **Hep.s.**
NOISE, CRACKING: **Bar.c.**
NOISE, LIKE BELLS RINGING: **Led.**

OTITIS MEDIA: **Bell.**
OTORRHOEA FOETID: **Aur.**
OTORRHOEA MUCO-PURULENT: **Calc.c.**
OTORRHOEA OBSTINATE: **Aur.**

PAIN CAUSES DELIRIUM: **Bell.**
PAIN CHILD CRIES IN SLEEP: **Bell.**

REDNESS: **Agar.**
REDNESS AND SORENESS BEHIND: **Petr.**
RINGING IN: **China.**
ROARING IN: **Led.; Lyc.; Merc.s.; Nit.a.; Petr.**

SENSITIVE TO LOUD SOUNDS: **Sil.**
SENSITIVE TO NOISE: **Acon.**
STOPPED UP FEELING: **Merc.s.**

TEARING STITCH, LEFT EAR: **Staph.**

WHIZZING IN: **Petr.**

NOSE

CATARRH, CHRONIC: Nat.c.; Spig.; Thuj.
CATARRH, DRY: Nux v.; Sul.
CATARRH, GREEN: Thuj.
CATARRH, THICK: Thuj.
CATARRH, VIOLENT: Lyc.
COLD AT EVERY CHANGE IN WEATHER: Calc.c.
COLDNESS, ICY, TIP OF: Ver.a.
CORYZA, DRY: Amm.c.
CORYZA, FLUENT IN DAYTIME: Nux v.
CORYZA, WITH HOARSENESS: Caust.

DISCHARGE, ACRID: Amm.m.
DISCHARGE, ACRID CORRODING UPPER LIP: All.c.
DISCHARGE, CORROSIVE: Nit.a.
DISCHARGE, FROM BOTH NOSTRILS: Nux v.
DISCHARGE, LARGE GREEN PLUGS: Sep.
DISCHARGE, OF MUCUS: Agar.
DISCHARGE, OFFENSIVE: Hep.s.
DISCHARGE, SMELLS LIKE OLD CHEESE: Hep.s.
DISCHARGE, STRINGY: Kali b.
DISCHARGE, THICK: Alum.; Hep.s.
DISCHARGE, TOUGH: Kali b.
DISCHARGE, WATERY: Amm.m.
DISCHARGE, YELLOW: Alum.
DISCHARGE, YELLOW/GREEN: Nat.s.

FAN-LIKE MOTION OF ALAE NASI: Lyc.

HAY-FEVER: Hep.s.; Lach.

ITCHING, VIOLENT: Nit.a.

MUCUS: Rhus t.
MUCUS FROM ONE NOSTRIL: Phyt.
MUCUS YELLOW: Puls.

NASAL BONE PAINFUL: Merc.s.
NOSE DRY: Acon.
NOSE ITCHING INSIDE AND OUTSIDE: Agar.
NOSE NERVOUS MOVEMENTS OF: Agar.

NOSE OBSTRUCTED: Amm.m.
NOSE PAIN AT ROOT OF: Acon.; Agar.
NOSE PAINFUL: Aur.
NOSE POINT OF, CRACKED: Alum.
NOSE PRESSURE AT ROOT OF: Kali b.
NOSE REDNESS: Alum.
NOSE SENSITIVE TO SMELL: Acon.
NOSE STOPPAGE AT NIGHT: Acon.
NOSE STOPPED UP: Lyc.
NOSE STOPPED UP SENSATION: Acon.
NOSE STUFFED UP IN WARM ROOM: Kali c.
NOSE STUFFED UP WITH DRYNESS AND BURNING: Nat.s.
NOSE STUFFED UP WHEN THERE IS COLD RAIN: Dulc.
NOSE STUFFY FEELING: Amm.m.
NOSE, SWELLING OF: Bar.c.
NOSE, ULCERATED: Aur.
NOSE BLEEDS: Bell.; Nit.a.; Phos.; Puls.; Sul.
NOSE BLEEDS AFTER EATING: Amm.c.
NOSE BLEEDS CANNOT BREATHE THROUGH: Amm.c.
NOSE BLEEDS DAILY, WITH PALE FACE: Carb.v.
NOSE BLEEDS DURING SLEEP: Merc.s.
NOSE BLEEDS IN OLD PEOPLE: Agar.
NOSE BLEEDS WHEN WASHING FACE: Amm.c.
NOSTRILS BURNING: Petr.
NOSTRILS CHAPPED: Ant.c.
NOSTRILS CRACKED: Ant.c.; Petr.
NOSTRILS CRUSTS, COVERED WITH: Ant.c.
NOSTRILS SCABBY: Sep.; Sul.
NOSTRILS SCURFY: Ant.c.
NOSTRILS SORE: Ant.c.; Calc.c.; Sep.
NOSTRILS SWOLLEN: Sep.
NOSTRILS ULCERATED: Calc.c.; Kali c.; Nit.a.; Petr.; Sep.;
Thuj.

ODOUR OFFENSIVE: Merc.s.

PAIN PRESSING, AT ROOT OF: Puls.; Thuj.
PIMPLES: Caust.
POLIPI: Cal.c.; Calc.p.
PUS GREEN, FOETID: Merc.'s.

SEPTUM ULCERATED: Kali b.
SMELL, LOSS OF: Amm.m.; Kali b.

SMELL, PUTRID: **Aur.**
SNEEZING AFTER SLEEP: **Lach.**
SNEEZING DRY: **China.**
SNEEZING FREQUENT: **All.c.; Bar.c.; Merc.s.; Nux v.; Rhus t.**
SNEEZING SPASMODIC: **Rhus t.**
SNEEZING VIOLENT: **China.; Kali b; Nat.m.; Rhus t.**
SNORING, DEEP: **Op.**
SNUFFLES IN CHILDREN: **Amm.c.**

TOUGH ELASTIC PLUGS: **Kali b.**

WARTS: **Caust.**

YELLOW SADDLE ACROSS NOSE: **Sep.**

FACE

BESOTTED: **Bapt.; Gels.**
BLUE: **Ver.a.**
BLUISH-RED: **Bell.**

CHEEKS, ERUPTIONS YELLOW, CRUSTED: **Ant.c.**
CHEEKS, ONE COLD AND PALE, THE OTHER RED
HOT: **Cham.**
CHEEKS, PAIN, TEARING TO RIGHT EAR: **Dulc.**
CHEEKS, PAIN, TEARING TO RIGHT EYE: **Dulc.**
CHEEKS, PAIN, TEARING TO RIGHT JAW: **Dulc.**
COBWEBS, FEELING OF: **Graph.**
COLD: **Ver.a.**
COLDNESS, ICY: **Ver.a.**
COLLAPSED: **Ver.a.**

DARK: **Op.**
DEATHLY PALE ON RISING: **Acon.**
DUSKY: **Bapt.**

EXPRESSION OF TERROR: **Stram.**

FLUSHED: **Bapt.; Ferr.m.; Gels.; Op.; Phyt.**

GREASY: **Plumb.**

HOT: **Arn.; Bapt.; Gels.; Op.; Stram.**

LIPS CRACKED: **Bry.**
LIPS DRY: **Bry.**
LIPS PARCHED: **Bry.**
LIPS SWELLING OF UPPER: **Bar.c.**

MUSCLES STIFF: **Agar.**
MUSCLES TWITCHING: **Agar.**

NEURALGIA OF: **Acon.**
NEURALGIA WITH NUMBNESS: **Acon.**
NEURALGIA WITH PAINS, PAROXYSMS: **Colo.**
NEURALGIA WITH PAINS, TEARING: **Colo.**
NEURALGIA WITH PAINS, TINGLING, SEVERE: **Acon.**

NEURALGIA WITH PAINS, VIOLENT: Colo.
NEURALGIA WORSE EXPOSURE TO COLD: Dulc.

PALE: Op.; Plumb.; Sep.; Ver.a.
PALE COVERED WITH SWEAT: Ant.t.

QUIVERING OF CHIN: Ant.t.
QUIVERING OF LOWER JAW: Ant.t.

RED, DARK: Bapt.; Stram.
RED, DURING CHILL: Ferr.m.
RED, FIERY: Ferr.m.
SUFFUSED: Op.
SWOLLEN: Op.
YELLOW: Plumb.; Sep.

MOUTH

APHTHOUS SORE: Bor.

BLISTERS ON SIDE OF: Thuj.
BLUE LINE ALONG MARGIN OF GUMS: Plumb.
BREATH OFFENSIVE: Kali p.
BURNING: Canth.

CANCER SORES: Ant.c.
COLD SORES ROUND: Hep.s.; Nat.m.
COMPLAINTS OF TEETHING CHILDREN: Mag.p.
CONTRACTION OF JAWS: Cup.m.
CORNERS OF MOUTH ULCERATED: Mers.s.; Nit.a.
CRACKS IN CORNERS: Ant.c.; Nit.a.
CRACKS IN MIDDLE OF LOWER LIP: Puls.

DESIRE TO PRESS GUMS TOGETHER: Pod.
DRYNESS: Acon.; Bry.; Kali p.; Phos.ac.; Puls.

FOAMS AT: Hyper.

GLAIRY SALIVA DRIBBLING FROM: Stram.
GUMS SENSITIVE TO COLD WATER: Sil.
GUMS SPONGY: Nit.a.
GUMS ULCERATED: Nit.a.

HAWKING OF THICK MUCUS: Nat.c.
HICCOUGH: Merc.s.
HOT: Bor.

JAW CRACKING WHILE EATING: Lac.c.

LIPS BRIGHT RED: Sul.
LIPS BURNING: Sul.
LOCKJAW: Nux v.

PALATE SENSITIVE: Nat.s.
SALIVA SWEET: Puls.
SALIVA WITH CONSTANT NAUSEA AND VOMITING: Ipec.
SMELL, FOUL FROM: Nit.a.; Spig.
SPITTING OF THICK MUCUS: Nat.c.

STAMMERS: Stram.
SWELLING OF: Merc.s.

TASTE, BAD: Puls.
TASTE, BITTER: Colo.; Nat.s.; Nux v.; Puls.; Sil.
TASTE, BURNT, AS IF: Bapt.; Puls.
TASTE, DIMINISHED: Puls.
TASTE, DRY: Bry.
TASTE, FOUL: Puls.
TASTE, GREASY: Puls.
TASTE, LOSS OF: Nat.m.
TASTE, METALLIC: Cup.m.
TASTE, PUTRID: Nux v.
TASTE, ROTTEN EGGS, OF: Arn.; Merc.s.
TASTE, SALTY: Merc.s.; Puls.
TASTE, SLIMY: Merc.s.
TASTE, SOUR: Merc.s.
TASTE, SOUR PERSISTENT: Calc.c.
TEETH ACHE: Staph.
TEETH ACHE BETTER ICE-COLD WATER: Coff.; Ferr.m.
TEETH ACHE WORSE AFTER WARM DRINK: Cham.
TEETH BLACK: Staph.
TEETH CRUMBLING: Staph.
TEETH GRINDING OF: Bell.
TEETH LOOSE: Merc.s.
TEETHING, SLOWNESS OF: Calc.p.
THIRST FOR COLD MILK: Phos.ac.
THIRST FOR COLD DRINKS: Nat.s.
THIRST FOR LARGE QUANTITIES OF COLD WATER: Acon.
THIRST FOR LONG DRINKS, EXCESSIVE: Bry.
THIRST UNQUENCHABLE: Nat.m.; Op.
THIRST VIOLENT: Merc.s.
TONGUE, BLISTERS ON: Lyc.; Nat.m.
TONGUE, BROAD: Pod.
TONGUE, BROWN, BITTER COATING: Nat.c.
TONGUE, BURNING: Nat.s.; Pod.
TONGUE, CLEAN WITH NAUSEA: Ipec.; Nit.a.
TONGUE, CRACKED: Hyos.
TONGUE, DRY: Hyos.; Kali b.; Lach.; Rhus t.; Stram.
TONGUE, GLAZED: Kali b.
TONGUE, HARD: Hyos.
TONGUE, LARGE: Pod.
TONGUE, MAPPED: Nat.m.

TONGUE, MOIST: **Pod.**
TONGUE, NUMB: **Nat.m.**
TONGUE, PARALYSED, FEELS: **Plumb.**
TONGUE, PARALYSIS OF: **Op.**
TONGUE, PARCHED, WHITE: **Hyos.**
TONGUE, RED: **Kali b.; Nit.a.**
TONGUE, SORE: **Rhus t.**
TONGUE, STIFFNESS OF: **Lac.c.**
TONGUE, STREAKED DOWN THE MIDDLE: **Bapt.**
TONGUE, TENACIOUS MUCUS, COVERED WITH: **Puls.**
TONGUE, THICK, WHITE COATING: **Ant.c.; Ant.t.**
TONGUE, TIP OF, RED: **Phyt.**
TONGUE, TREMBLES: **Lach.; Plumb.**
TONGUE, ULCERATED: **Bapt.**
TONGUE, WET: **Nit.a.**
TONGUE, WHITE: **Acon.; Merc.s.; Puls.**
TONGUE, YELLOW: **Kali b.; Puls.**
TONGUE, YELLOW–RED MARGINS SHOWING IMPRINT OF
TEETH: **Chel.**
TWITCHING MUSCLES OF FACE: **Ign.**
TWITCHING MUSCLES OF LIPS: **Ign.**

ULCERS IN SOFT PALATE: **Nit.a.**

WATER IN, AT NIGHT: **Merc.s.**

YAWNING, SPASMODIC: **Rhus t.**
YAWNING, VIOLENT: **Rhus t.**

THROAT

ADENOIDS: Calc.p.

BLUISH-RED: Phyt.
BURNING: Amm.m.; Canth.
BURNING LIKE FIRE: Bell.

CERVICAL MUSCLES TWITCHING: Agar.
CHOKING SENSATION: Lach.
CONSTRICTION OF: Stram.
CONSTRICTION, FEELING OF: Bell.
CRAWLING IN, WHICH PROVOKES COUGHING: Dros.

DARK: Phyt.
DEGLUTITION DIFFICULT: Bell.
DIPHTHERIA: Lach.
DRY: Acon.; Alum.; Puls.; Rhus t.; Stram.

FOLLICULAR TONSILLITIS: Ign.

GLANDS ENLARGED: Rhus t.
GLANDS INGUINAL, INFLAMED: Merc.s.
GLANDS INGUINAL, PAINFUL: Merc.s.
GLANDS INGUINAL, RED: Merc.s.
GLANDS INGUINAL, SWOLLEN: Merc.s.
GLANDS NAPE OF NECK SWOLLEN: Bar.c.
GLANDS NECK, SWOLLEN: Bar.c.

HOARSENESS: All.c.; Amm.m.; Bell.; Petr.; Phos.ac.; Spong.
HOT: Phyt.

INFLAMMATION: Lyc.

LARYNX, BURNING: Spong.
LARYNX, DRY: Spong.
LARYNX, FEELS TORN: All.c.
LARYNX, RAW: Cham.; Nux v.; Phos.
LARYNX, TICKLES: All.c.
LARYNX, TICKLING FROM COUGH: Nit.a.

MUCUS TENACIOUS, VERY: Canth.

MUCUS THICK: Arg.n.

NAPE OF NECK ACHING: Zinc.
NAPE WEARINESS IN: Zinc.
NECK, NEURALGIC PAIN SEVERE: Mag.p.
NECK, STIFFNESS OF: Lac.c.

PAIN SHOOTING INTO EARS ON SWALLOWING: Phyt.
PAIN SMARTING: Bar.c.
PAIN STICKING: Kali c.; Nit.a.
PAIN STINGING: Bar.c.; Nit.a.
PAINFUL: Bell.; Puls.
PALATE, SOFT SWOLLEN: Bapt.
PARALYSIS OF: Gels.
PUFFY: Mag.p.

QUINSY: Hep.s.

RED: Bell.
ROUGH: Phyt.
ROUGH FROM CATARRH: Nux v.
ROUGH SCRAPING DEEP DOWN: Dros.

SCRATCHY: Puls.
SENSATION OF DRY FEATHERY DUST: Ign.
SENSATION OF SPLINTER IN THROAT WHEN
SWALLOWING: Arg.n.; Hep.s.
SORE: Nit.a.; Puls.
SPASMS IN: Bell.
STITCHES FLY FROM THROAT TO EAR: Staph.
STRANGLED FEELING: Arg.n.
SWALLOW, INABILITY TO: Hyos.
SWALLOW, ONLY LIQUIDS: Bapt.; Bar.c.
SWALLOWING DIFFICULT: Nit.a.
SWALLOWING DIFFICULT WITH LIQUIDS: Canth.
SWALLOWING SOLIDS BETTER THAN EMPTY
SWALLOWING: Lach.
SWELLING WITH VISCID PHLEGM: Amm.m.
SWOLLEN: Nit.a.; Rhus t.
SYMPTOMS KEEP CHANGING: Lac.c.
SYMPTOMS WORSE HOT DRINKS: Lach.

TONSILS ENLARGED: Bell.; Calc.p.

TONSILS INFLAMED: Ign.
TONSILS SUPPURATING: Bar.c.
TONSILS SWOLLEN: Bapt.; Bar.c.; Calc.c.; Ign.; Phyt.
TONSILS ULCERATION OF: Lyc.
TOUCHED, CANNOT BEAR THROAT TO BE: Lach.

ULCERATION: Lach.; Nit.a.
UVULA ELONGATED: Hyos.

VOICE HARSH: Ant.c.
VOICE HAWKING: Cham.
VOICE HOARSENESS: Cham
VOICE HOARSENESS WORSE EVENING: Carb.v.
VOICE HUSKY: Phos.
VOICE LOSS OF: Caust.
VOICE PIPING, HIGH: Bell.
VOICE PITCHED BADLY: Ant.c.
VOICE PITCHED HIGH: Bell.

WHITE PATCHES ON: Nit.a.

STOMACH

ACIDITY IN: Sul.
ANXIETY IN: Kali c.
APPETITE, LOSS OF: Ant.t.; Plumb.
APPETITE, LOSS OF WHEN OVERWORKED: Calc.c.
APPETITE VORACIOUS: Ferr.m.; Ver.a.
AVERSION TO DRINK: Dulc.
AVERSION TO FATS: Carb.v.; Puls.
AVERSION TO FOOD: Dulc.
AVERSION TO TOBACCO: Dulc.
AVERSION TO WARM DRINKS: Puls.
AVERSION TO WARM FOOD: Puls.

BELCHING ACCOMPANIES MOST AILMENTS: Arg.n.
BELCHING CONSTANT: Ant.c.
BLOATED FEELING AFTER EATING: Ant.c.
BREAD DISAGREES: Nit.a.
BURNING CAUSES HUNGER: Graph.
BURNING IN PIT OF STOMACH: Sep.
BURNING SENSATION: Canth.
BURNING VIOLENT, OCCASIONAL: Colch.

COLD FEELING IN: Ver.a.
COLD SENSITIVE TO: Colo.
COLIC, FLATULENT: Cham.; China.; Mag.p.; Nat.s.
COLIC, FLATULENT WORSE AFTER SUPPER: Puls.
COLIC, PAINTER'S: Op.
COLIC, VIOLENT: Op.
CONTRACTION IN: Plumb.
CRAVES BACON: Calc.p.
CRAVES HAM: Calc.p.
CRAVES INDIGESTIBLE THINGS: Calc.c.
CRAVES SALT: Nat.m.
CRAVES SALTED MEATS: Calc.p.
CRAVES SMOKED MEATS: Calc.p.
CRAVES TOBACCO: Staph.
CRAVES VARIOUS FOODS NOT WANTED WHEN
COOKED: Colch.

DESIRES ACID FOOD: Ant.c.; Ant.t.
DESIRES APPLES: Ant.t.

DESIRES FRUITS: Ant.t.
DESIRES PICKLES: Ant.c.
DIGESTION WEAK: Nat.s.
DISLIKES FAT: Calc.c.
DISTENDED: Amb.g.; Bar.c.
DISTENTION PAINFUL: Lach.; Thuj.
DISTURBED EASILY BY CAKES: Puls.
DISTURBED EASILY BY FAT: Puls.
DISTURBED EASILY BY PASTRY: Puls.
DISTURBED EASILY BY RICH FOOD: Puls.
DRINK, CONSTANT DESIRE TO: Colo.
DRINK, COLD, LONGS FOR: Calc.c.
DRINKING COFFEE, WORSE FOR: Canth.
DRINKING DREADS: Bell
DRINKING WHEN, LIQUID DESCENDS WITH GURGLING
SOUND: Cup.m.

EATING AFTER, DISTENTION: Kali c.
EATING AFTER, FULLNESS: Kali c.
EATING AFTER, HEAT: Kali c.
EATING, VERY LITTLE CREATES FULLNESS: Lyc.
EMPTY FEELING IN: Anac.; Sep.
ERUCTATIONS AFTER A MEAL: Ferr.m.
ERUCTATIONS EMPTY: Carb.v.
ERUCTATIONS FREQUENT: Puls.
ERUCTATIONS LIKE ROTTEN EGGS: Arn.
ERUCTATIONS SOUR: Calc.c.

FAINT FEELING: Sep.
FAINT FEELING ABOUT 11 a.m.: Sul.
FAINTNESS WHEN SITTING UP: Bry.
FLATULENCE: Calc.p.; Ign.; Kali c.; Lach.; Puls.; Thuj.
FLATUS PASSED WITH DIFFICULTY: Nat.s.
FOOD PUTRIFIES BEFORE IT DIGESTS: Carb.v.
FOOD TASTES SOUR: Lyc.
FULLNESS, FEELING OF: Carb.v.

GASTRITIS: Hyos.
GIDDY AFTER SLIGHT MEAL: Petr.
GRIPING AFTER EATING: Zinc.

HARD: Bar.c.
HEARTBURN: Calen.

HUNGER, EXTREME WHEN STOMACH FULL OF
FOOD: **Staph.**
HUNGER, GREAT: **Spong.**
HUNGER, RAVENOUS ABOUT 11 a.m.:   **Zinc.**

ICY COLDNESS IN: **Colch.**
INTOLERANCE OF EGGS: **Ferr.m.**

LOVES FAT: **Nit.a.**
LOVES SALT: **Nit.a.**

MILK DISAGREES: **Sul.**

NAUSEA: **Ant.t.; Chel.; Hyper.; Ipec.; Plumb.; Ver.a.**
NAUSEA AFTER A MEAL: **Nux v.**
NAUSEA AFTER EATING: **Sep.**
NAUSEA AFTER WAKING: **Petr.**
NAUSEA ALL DAY: **Petr.**
NAUSEA BEFORE BREAKFAST: **Berb.**
NAUSEA FROM RIDING IN A VEHICLE: **Sep.**
NAUSEA FROM SITTING UP: **Bry.**
NAUSEA FROM SMELL OF COOKING: **Colch.; Sep.**
NAUSEA FROM SMELL OF FOOD: **Colch.**
NAUSEA MORNING: **Nux v.; Sep.**
NAUSEA SUDDEN WITH WATER IN MOUTH: **Petr.**

PAIN BETTER DRINK: **Graph.**
PAIN BETTER EATING: **Anac.**
PAIN BETTER FOOD: **Graph.**
PAIN BETTER LYING DOWN: **Graph.**
PAIN CONSTRICTIVE: **Graph.**
PAIN CONTRACTIVE: **Carb.v.**
PAIN GNAWING: **Cimic.**
PAIN ONLY WHEN STOMACH IS EMPTY: **Anac.**
PAIN WITH CLEAN TONGUE: **Mag.p.**
PRESSURE IN: **Phos.**
PRESSURE IN AFTER EATING: **Bry.; Phos.ac.**
PRESSURE IN AFTER EATING LITTLE: **Nux v.**

REGURGITATION OF FOOD IMMEDIATELY AFTER
MEAL: **Ferr.m.**
RETCHING: **Ant.t.**

SENSATION AS IF HANGING DOWN: **Staph.**
SENSATION OF SICKNESS: **Puls.**
SENSITIVE: **Canth.**
SHIVERY AND CHILLY WITHOUT THIRST: **Staph.**
SICKNESS AFTER MEAL: **Nux v.**
SICKNESS OF PREGNANCY, MORNING: **Sep.**
SICKNESS SEA: **Petr.**
SINKING FEELING IN: **Bapt.**
SPITS UP FOOD BY MOUTHFULS: **Colch.**
SWEATING: **Acon.**
SWEATING WHILE EATING: **Nat.m.**
SWELLING, PIT OF, PAINFUL: **Arg.n.**

TENSION IN: **Ruta.**
THIRST FOR COLD DRINKS: **Dulc.**
THIRST FOR COLD WATER: **Ant.t.; Bell.**
THIRST FOR COLD WATER VOMITED WHEN
SWALLOWED: **Ver.a.**

ULCER, ROUND: **Kali b.**
ULCERATION OF, WITH RADIATING PAINS: **Arg.n.**

VOMITS: **Ant.t.; Ver.a.**
VOMITS INCLINATION TO: **Puls.**
VOMITS WITH FEAR: **Acon.**
VOMITING AFTER EATING (IMMEDIATELY):   **Ferr.m.**
VOMITING AFTER MIDNIGHT: **Ferr.m.**
VOMITING BETTER DRINKING VERY HOT WATER: **Chel.**
VOMITING OF BILE: **Nat.s.**
VOMITING OF FOOD: **Phos.**
VOMITING OF GREEN BILE: **Stram.**
VOMITING OF MUCUS: **Stram.**
VOMITING ROPY: **Kali b.**
VOMITING SOUR: **Calc.c.**
VOMITING WITH NAUSEA: **Ipec.**

WINE, SMALLEST AMOUNT UPSETS: **Zinc.**

ABDOMEN

ABDOMINAL WALL FEELS DRAWN BY STRING TO
SPINE: **Plumb.**

BLOATED: **Lyc.; Mag.p.**

CHOLERA INFANTUM: **Zinc.**
COLD FEELING IN: **Ver.a.**
COLIC: **Plumb.**
COLIC CAUSING NAUSEA: **Nux v.**
COLIC FLATULENT: **Carb.v.; Cham.**
COLIC RADIATING TO ALL PARTS: **Plumb.**
COMPLAINTS LEFT SIDED: **Alum.**
CONTRACTED, FEELS: **Cup.m.**

DISTENDED AFTER EATING: **Kali c.**
DISTENDED WITH WIND AND FEELS FULL OF SHARP
STONES: **Cocc.**
DISTENSION: **Amb.g.; Carb.v.; China.; Colch.; Lyc.; Sep.; Stram.**
DISTENSION FLATULENT: **Nux v.**
DISTENSION WITH HARDNESS: **Calc.c.**

FEELS WEAK AND EMPTY: **Phos.**
FLABBY: **Calc.p.**
FLATULENCE: **Nit.a.**
FLATULENCE INCARCERATED: **Graph.**
FLATUS OBSTRUCTED, WITH PAINFUL COLIC: **Plumb.**

GLANDS, INGUINAL, PAINFUL: **Calc.c.**
GLANDS, INGUINAL, SWOLLEN: **Calc.c.**
GLANDS, MESENTERIC, PAINFUL: **Calc.c.**
GLANDS, MESENTERIC, SWOLLEN: **Calc.c.**

HARD: **Sil.**

JAUNDICE: **Nit.a.; Pod.**

MUSCLES OF, ACUTELY PAINFUL: **Bapt.**
MUSCLES OF, SORE ON PRESSING: **Bapt.**

PAINS, ACHING IN HEPATIC REGION: **Ruta.**

PAINS, AGONIZING, CAUSING PATIENT TO BEND
DOUBLE: Colo.
PAINS, AROUND LIVER: Pod.
PAINS, BURNING, WORSE BREATHING: Bry.
PAINS, BURNING, WORSE COUGHING: Bry.
PAINS, BURNING, WORSE PRESSURE: Bry.
PAINS, COLICKY ON EATING: Calc.p.
PAINS, CUTTING, CAUSING PATIENT TO BEND
DOUBLE: Colo.
PAINS, CUTTING, WITH DISCHARGE OF FLATUS: Puls.
PAINS, IN ABDOMINAL RING, FEELS AS THOUGH
SOMETHING IS PUSHED THROUGH: Cocc.
PAINS, STICKING, AROUND LIVER: Nat.s.
PAINS, STITCHING: Bry.
PRESSURE, AS THOUGH CONTENTS WOULD DROP
THROUGH GENITAL ORGANS: Sep.

RUMBLING: Nit.a.; Phos.ac.; Sep.

SENSATION AS IF HANGING DOWN: Staph.
SENSATION OF EMPTINESS: Sep.
SENSATION OF SINKING: Pod.
SENSITIVITY OF LIVER AREA: Nat.s.
SPOTS, DARK BROWN, LIVER: Plumb.
SUNKEN: Calc.p.

TENDER, EXTREMELY: Apis.
TENSE: Sil.
TENSION IN LIVER AREA: Nat.s.

WEAKNESS OF: Pod.
WRITHES IN AGONY: Colo.

Rectum

ANUS, BURNING IN: Op.
ANUS, CRACKED: Nit.a.
ANUS, ECZEMA AROUND: Graph.
ANUS, FISSURED: Nit.a.
ANUS, ITCHING OF: Anac.
ANUS, OPEN, SEEMS: Anac.
ANUS, REDNESS AROUND: Sul.
ANUS, SENSATION OF PLUG IN: Anac.

BOWELS, RUMBLE: Bapt.
BURNING: Sil.

CONSTIPATION: Amm.m.; Nat.m.
CONSTIPATION ALMOST INCURABLE: Op.
CONSTIPATION DURING PREGNANCY: Sep.
CONSTRICTION AFTER STOOL: Ign.
CONSTRICTION DRAWN UP WITH: Plumb.

DIARRHOEA AFTER HUNGER: Petr.
DIARRHOEA ALTERNATES WITH CONSTIPATION: Ant.c.;
Chel.
DIARRHOEA BLACK: Plumb.
DIARRHOEA CHRONIC: Nat.m.; Nit.a.
DIARRHOEA CREAM COLOURED: Gels.
DIARRHOEA DAYTIME, IN: Petr.
DIARRHOEA EARLY MORNING: Pod.
DIARRHOEA FROM EMOTIONAL EXCITEMENT: Gels.
DIARRHOEA GREEN (TEA): Gels.
DIARRHOEA IN MORNING: Sul.
DIARRHOEA INVOLUNTARY: Hyos.
DIARRHOEA LUMPY: Plumb.
DIARRHOEA OF CHILDREN: Calc.c.; Pod.
DIARRHOEA WATERY: Phos.ac.
DIARRHOEA WHITE: Phos.ac.
DIARRHOEA WITH FOUL, PUTRID ODOUR: Kali p.
DIARRHOEA WITHOUT DEBILITY: Phos.ac.
DIARRHOEA WITHOUT PAIN: Phos.ac.
DIARRHOEA YELLOW: Phos.ac.
DISCHARGE YELLOW: Nat.c.

FISSURE IN: Graph.
FISSURED: Thuj.
FISTULA IN ANO: Berb.
FLATUS HOT: Staph.
FLATUS OFFENSIVE: Sil.

HAEMORRHOIDS, BLIND: Nux v.
HAEMORRHOIDS, PAINFUL: Sil
HAEMORRHOIDS, PAINFUL ACHING: Lyc.; Nit.a.

INACTIVE: Alum.

MOISTURE IN: Anac.
MOISTURE ACRID, FROM: Carb.v.
MOISTURE CORROSIVE: Carb.v.

PAIN AFTER STOOL: Carb.v.
PAINS AFTER STOOL LAST FOR HOURS: Nit.a.
PAINS SHARP AFTER STOOL: Nux v.
PILES, BLEEDING: Hyper.
PILES, BLUISH: Carb.v.
PILES, BURNING: Carb.v.
PRESSURE FROM WITHIN/OUTWARDS, AS FROM SHARP
INSTRUMENT: Ign.
PROLAPSE: Ign.; Pod.

REMAINS, FEELS AS THOUGH SOMETHING STAYS BEHIND
AFTER STOOL: Nux v.

SPASM OF: Plumb.
STOOL, BLACK BALLS: Op.
STOOL, BLOODY: Bapt.
STOOL, BLOODY MUCUS: Dulc.
STOOL, CLOTS, DARK: China.
STOOL, COLD SWEAT: Ver.a.
STOOL, CRUMBLING: Amm.m.; Nat.m.
STOOL, DARK: Sil.
STOOL, DESIRE FOR, BUT INSUFFICIENT ACTION: Anac.
STOOL, DESIRE NONE: Alum.
STOOL, DIFFICULT: Amm.m.; Ign.; Lach.; Lyc.; Sil.
STOOL, DRY: Amm.m.; Sil.
STOOL, FLATUS FOETID: Calc.p.
STOOL, FOETID: Cham.; Hep.s.; Pod.
STOOL, FROTHY: China.; Op.

STOOL, GREEN: Arg.n.; Calc.p.; Cham.; Dulc.; Pod.

STOOL, GUSHING: Pod.

STOOL, HARD: Alum.; Amm.m.; Lyc.; Nat.m.; Op.; Plumb.; Sil.

STOOL, HARD WITH WATERY DISCHARGE: Ant.c.

STOOL, HOT: Calc.p.; Cham.

STOOL, INVOLUNTARY: Op.; Phos.ac.

STOOL, JELLY-LIKE: Colo.

STOOL, KNOTTY: Alum.; Graph.

STOOL, LARGE: Graph.; Ver.a.

STOOL, LOOSE: Nat.s.

STOOL, MUCUS: Bor.

STOOL, MUCUS LIKE SCRAPING OF INTESTINE: Canth.

STOOL, OFFENSIVE: Bapt.; Graph.; Lach.

STOOL, PAINFUL: Lach.

STOOL, PAINLESS: China.

STOOL, PROFUSE: Pod.

STOOL, REMAINS LONG IN RECTUM: Sil.

STOOL, ROTTEN EGGS, LIKE: Arn.

STOOL, ROUND: Op.

STOOL, SHEEP'S DUNG, LIKE: Alum.

STOOL, SHIVERING WITH: Canth.

STOOL, SHUDDERING WITH: Canth.

STOOL, SLIMY: Calc.p.; Cham.; Dulc.

STOOL, SLIPS BACK, MAY: Sil.

STOOL, SOFT: Bor.

STOOL, SOFT PASSED WITH GREAT DIFFICULTY: Alum.

STOOL, SOUR: Calc.c.; Hep.s.

STOOL, SPLUTTERING: Calc.p.

STOOL, STOMACH-ACHE, AFTER: Puls.

STOOL, SUDDEN CALL TO: Nat.c.

STOOL, THIN: Bapt.

STOOL, UNDIGESTED: China.; Hep.s.

STOOL, UNDIGESTED PAINLESS AT NIGHT: Ferr.m.

STOOL, WATERY: Cham.; Dulc.; Pod.

STOOL, WHITE: Hep.s.; Puls.

STOOL, WITH COLIC: Cham.

STOOL, YELLOW: China.; Puls.

STOOL, YELLOW, LIGHT: Bor.

URGING FOR STOOL WITH RARE EVACUATION: Hyos.

URGING FREQUENT AND INEFFECTUAL: Nux v.

WARTS ON AND AROUND: Thuj.

BED-WETTING: Sul.

BLADDER, IRRITABLE, IN YOUNG MARRIED WOMEN: Staph.

FLUIDS RUN RIGHT THROUGH HIM: Arg.n.

NEPHRITIS, CHRONIC: Plumb.

ODOUR OFFENSIVE: Nit.a.

RENAL COLIC: Lyc.

URGING, BUT SCANTY: Phos.ac.

URINE, CANNOT PASS WHEN ANYBODY ELSE IN
ROOM: Amb.g.; Nat.m.

URINE, COLD ON PASSING: Nit.a.

URINE, DRIBBLES WHEN SITTING: Puls.

URINE, FREQUENT: Bell.; Puls.

URINE, HOT: Acon.

URINE, MUCUS IN: Plumb.; Sul.

URINE, PAINFUL: Acon.

URINE, PALE BUT FORMS THICK, WHITE CLOUD: Phos.ac.

URINE, PASSED DROP BY DROP: Canth.

URINE, PROFUSE: Bell.; Gels.

URINE, PUS IN: Sil.

URINE, RETENTION OF: Acon.; Gels.

URINE, RETENTION BUT INVOLUNTARY AFTER
FRIGHT: Op.

URINE, RETENTION SCREAMS FREQUENTLY WHEN
PASSING: Bor.

URINE, SCANTY: Acon.

URINE, SCALDS: Canth.

URINE, SLOW IN STARTING: Lyc.

URINE, SUDDEN: Sul.

URINE, SUPPRESSED: Stram.

URINE, SUPPRESSED WITH PAIN IN KIDNEY REGION: Phyt.

URINE, TURBID: Amb.g.

URINE, WATERY: Gels.

URINE, YELLOW: Kali p.

URINATE, CONSTANT DESIRE: Canth.; Merc.s.

URINATE, FREQUENT CALL T,O, BUT LITTLE PASSED: Staph.

URINATE, FREQUENT PAINFUL INEFFECTUAL DESIRE
TO: Nux.v.

URINATE, INEFFECTUAL URGING IN NEWLY MARRIED
WOMEN: Staph.

URINATE, MUST, WHEN GETTING CHILLED: Dulc.

URINATE, URGING INTOLERABLE: **Canth.**
URINATING, AFTER, FEELS A FEW DROPS REMAIN: **Kali b.**
URINATING, WORSE BEFORE: **Bor.**
URINATION, INVOLUNTARY: **Hyos.; Nat.m.**

FEMALE

ABSCESS OF BREAST: **Phyt.**
ABSCESS OF LABIA: **Hep.s.**
AVERSION TO MOTHER'S MILK: **Sil.**

BREASTS HARD: **Phyt.; Sil.**
BREASTS PAINFUL: **Phyt.; Sil.**
BREASTS SWOLLEN, BETTER MENSES: **Lac.c.**
BREASTS SWOLLEN, (NIPPLE): **Sil.**
BREASTS ULCER, FISTULAR, IN: **Phyt.**

CLIMACTERIC, HOT, FLUSHED: **Sep.**

DYSMENORRHOEA: **Ver.a.**

FEELING AS IF VISCERA WOULD PROTRUDE: **Bell.**
FEELING OF FORCING DOWNWARDS: **Bell.**
FEMALE COMPLAINTS ASSOCIATED WITH COLDNESS: **Zinc.**
FEMALE COMPLAINTS ASSOCIATED WITH
DEPRESSION: **Zinc.**
FEMALE COMPLAINTS ASSOCIATED WITH
RESTLESSNESS: **Zinc.**
FEMALE COMPLAINTS ASSOCIATED WITH TENDER
SPINE: **Zinc.**
FEMALE COMPLAINTS BETTER MENSTRUAL FLOW: **Zinc.**

HAEMORRHAGE, PREVENTS: **Arn.**

LEUCORRHOEA, ACRID: **Alum.**
LEUCORRHOEA, BITING: **Merc.s.**
LEUCORRHOEA, EXCORIATING: **Graph.**
LEUCORRHOEA, GREENISH: **Merc.s.**
LEUCORRHOEA, GUSHING: **Cocc.**
LEUCORRHOEA, JELLY-LIKE: **Kali b.**
LEUCORRHOEA, PALE: **Graph.**
LEUCORRHOEA, PROFUSE: **Alum.; Graph.**
LEUCORRHOEA, PURULENT: **Cocc.**
LEUCORRHOEA, ROPY: **Alum.; Kali b.**
LEUCORRHOEA, SCANTY: **Ign.**
LEUCORRHOEA, THIN: **Graph.**

LEUCORRHOEA, WHITE: Graph.

LEUCORRHOEA, YELLOWISH/GREEN: Nat.s.

LEUCORRHOEA, BETWEEN MENSES, VERY
WEAKENING: Cocc.

MAMMARY GLANDS FULL OF HARD, PAINFUL
NODES: Phyt.

MAMMARY GLANDS INDURATION OF: Plumb.

MENSES, ACRID: Sul.

MENSES, BLACK: Sul.

MENSES, CEASE AT NIGHT, FLOW ONLY DAYTIME: Caust.

MENSES, CHANGEABLE: Puls.

MENSES, CLOTTED: Puls.

MENSES, WITH COLD, DAMP FEET: Calc.c.

MENSES, COAGULATED: Cimic.

MENSES, DARK: Cimic.; Puls.

MENSES, DEBILITATING: Ferr.m.

MENSES, BETWEEN DISCHARGE OF BLOOD: Amb.g.

MENSES, TOO EARLY: Bell.; Bor.; Calc.c.; Ferr.m.; Ign.

MENSES, TOO EARLY WITH CRAMPS: Nux v.

MENSES, WITH FIERY RED FACE: Ferr.m.

MENSES, FLOW IN GUSHES: Lac.c.

MENSES, FLOW MORE AT NIGHT: Amm.m.

MENSES, FLOW SCANTY: Gels.

MENSES, TOO FREQUENT: Amm.c.

MENSES, HOT: Bell.

MENSES, INCREASED: Bell.

MENSES, TOO LATE: Graph.; Kali p.; Sul.

MENSES, TOO LONG: Calc.c.; Ferr.m.

MENSES, OFFENSIVE, VERY: Bell.

MENSES, PAINFUL: Gels.

MENSES, PROFUSE: Amm.c.; Bell.; Berb.; Calc.c.; Cimic.;
Ferr.m.; Ign.

MENSES, RASH BEFORE THEY DEVELOP: Dulc.

MENSES, RED, BRIGHT: Bell.

MENSES, SCANTY: Alum.; Kali p.; Sul.

MENSES, SHORT: Sul.

MENSES, SUPPRESSED FROM FEAR: Acon.

MENSES, WITH TOOTHACHE: Calc.c.

MENSES, WITH VERTIGO: Calc.c.

MENSES, WATERY: Ferr.m.

MENSES, WEAKENING BETWEEN: Cocc.

MENSTRUAL COLIC: Mag.p.

MILK, HELPS TO DRY UP: Lac.c.

NAUSEA, MORNINGS DURING MENSES: Nux v.
NIPPLES CRACKED: Phyt.
NIPPLES EXCORIATED: Phyt.
NYMPHOMANIA: Canth.

PAIN IN OVARY, BORING: Colo.
PAIN OVARIAN: Zinc.
PAIN RIGHT OVARY: Pod.
PAIN ACROSS PELVIS, FROM HIP TO HIP: Cimic.
PAIN IN UTERUS: Pod.
PAINS, MUST DOUBLE UP: Colo.
PAINS, WITH GREAT RESTLESSNESS: Colo.
PELVIC ORGANS, SENSATION OF BEARING DOWN: Sep.
PROLAPSE, UTERUS: Aur.; Sep.
PROLAPSE, VAGINA: Ferr.m.; Sep.

SORENESS OF PARTS AFTER LABOUR: Arn.

UTERINE INERTIA DURING LABOUR: Caust.
UTERUS DISCHARGE PROFUSE, CLOTTED DARK BLOOD
WITH LABOUR-LIKE PAINS: Cham.
UTERUS ENLARGEMENT OF: Aur.
UTERUS PRESSURE AS THOUGH CONTENTS WOULD GO
THROUGH VULVA: Sep.

VAGINA BURNS: Sul.
VAGINA HYPERSENSITIVE: Coff.
VAGINISMUS: Plumb.
VOMITING IF CHILD IS NURSED: Sil.
VULVA HYPERSENSITIVE: Coff.

MALE

EMISSIONS FREQUENT: Calc.c.
ERECTIONS PAINFUL: Canth.

IMPOTENCE: Lyc.

PROSTATIC AFFECTIONS FROM SUPPRESSED
GONORRHOEA: Thuj.

RHEUMATISM, GONORRHOEAL: Thuj.

SEXUAL POWER, LOSS OF: Plumb.
SPERMATORRHOEA: Gels.

TESTICLES, ATROPHY OF, IN BOYS: Aur.

RESPIRATORY

ASTHMA: **Lach.**
ASTHMA IN CHILDREN: **Nat.s.**
ASTHMA IN THE AGED: **Carb.v.**
ASTHMA WHEN TALKING: **Dros.**
ASTHMA WITH BLUE SKIN: **Carb.v.**
ASTHMA WORSE FOG: **Hyper.**
ASTHMATIC BRONCHITIS: **Zinc.**

BREATH, SHORTNESS OF: **Spig.; Zinc.**
BREATHING DIFFICULT: **Acon.; Sul.**
BREATHING OPPRESSED FROM PRESSURE MID-CHEST: **All.c.**
BREATHING RAPID: **Op.**
BREATHING STERTOROUS: **Op.**
BREATHLESS, NIGHT, MUST SIT UP: **Sul.**
BREATHLESS, OPPRESSED: **Amm.c.**

CHEST, ANXIETY IN: **Phos.**
CHEST, CONSTRICTION IN: **Cact.; Ipec.; Led.**
CHEST, CONTRACTION OF: **Cup.m.**
CHEST, DRYNESS OF AIR PASSAGES: **Bry.**
CHEST, EMPHYSEMA FROM CHRONIC ASTHMA: **Ipec.**
CHEST, EMPHYSEMA IN OLD PEOPLE: **Ipec.**
CHEST, EXPECTORATION BLOODY WITH MUCUS: **Phos.**
CHEST, EXPECTORATION LITTLE BALLS OF MUCUS: **Agar.**
CHEST, EXPECTORATION SCANTY, MUST BE SWALLOWED: **Caust.**
CHEST, LUNG, OEDEMA OF: **Ant.t.**
CHEST, OPPRESSED: **Ferr.m.**
CHEST, OPPRESSION OF: **Lyc.; Nat.s.; Sul.**
CHEST, OPPRESSION OF SO THAT BREATH CANNOT BE EXPELLED: **Dros.**
CHEST, PAIN FROM WEAKNESS: **Phos.ac.**
CHEST, PAIN GNAWING LEFT SIDE: **Ruta.**
CHEST, PAIN PIERCING, LEFT SIDE WHEN BREATHING: **Nat.s.**
CHEST, PLEURISY WITH EXUDATION: **Canth.**
CHEST, PRESSURE ON: **Phos.; Nat.s.**
CHEST, RATTLING OF: **China.**

CHEST, RATTLING OF MUCUS: Sul.

CHEST, RATTLING OF MUCUS WITH LITTLE
EXPECTORATION: Ant.t.

CHEST, RAW, INTERNALLY: Lyc.

CHEST, SENSATION OF BURNING: Ant.c.

CHEST, SENSATION OF IRON BAND: Arg.n.; Cact.

CHEST, SENSATION OF SUFFOCATION WHEN
BREATHING: Bapt.

CHEST, SENSITIVE: Kali c.

CHEST, SENSITIVE TO PERCUSSION: Calc.c.

CHEST, SENSITIVE TO PRESSURE: Calc.c.

CHEST, SENSITIVE TO TOUCH: Calc.c.

CHEST, SPASMS IN: Cup.m.

CHEST, STITCHES IN LEFT SIDE ON INSPIRING: Lyc.

CHEST, SUFFOCATION, ATTACKS OF: Cact.

CHEST, SUFFOCATIVE CATARRH IN: China.

CHEST, SUFFOCATIVE FEELING AS IF HE COULD NOT
DRAW ANOTHER BREATH: Apis.

CHEST, SUFFOCATIVE SPELLS WORSE GOING UP
SLIGHTEST ASCENT: Calc.c.

CHEST, SUFFOCATIVE SPELLS WORSE GOING
UPSTAIRS: Calc.c.

CHEST, WEIGHT, FEELING OF, IN: Aur.

COUGH, BARKING: Amb.g.; Nit.a.; Spong.

COUGH, CAUSES HEADACHE: Nux v.

COUGH, CHOKING: Hep.s.

COUGH, CHRONIC: Nit.a.

COUGH, CROUP WORSE BEFORE MIDNIGHT: Spong.

COUGH, CROUP WORSE INSPIRING: Spong.

COUGH, CROUPY: Spong.

COUGH, DEEP, HOARSE, SPASMODIC UNTIL HE RETCHES
OR VOMITS: Dros.

COUGH, DRY: Acon.; Alum.; Bell.; Bry.; Cham.; Cimic.; Hyos.;
Kali c.; Nit.a.; Phos.; Spong.

COUGH, EXCITED BY TOUCHING THROAT: Lach.

COUGH, EXCITED ON UNCOVERING BODY: Hep.s.

COUGH, FROM IRRITATION BEHIND STERNUM: Rhus t.

COUGH, HACKING: All.c.; Alum.

COUGH, HARD: Kali c.

COUGH, HOARSE: Acon.

COUGH, HOLLOW: Amb.g.

COUGH, INCESSANT: Ipec.; Sep.

COUGH, IRRITABLE: Cham.

COUGH, LARYNGEAL: Nit.a.
COUGH, NERVOUS: Amb.g.
COUGH, NIGHT, WHEN LYING: Hyos.
COUGH, PHYSICAL EXERTION, AFTER: Dulc.
COUGH, SHORT: Bell.; Cimic.
COUGH, SINGING, WHEN: Alum.
COUGH, SLEEP, DURING: Lach.
COUGH, SNEEZE, ENDS IN: Agar.
COUGH, SPASMODIC: Amb.g.; Hyos.; Mag.p.
COUGH, SPASMS AFTER FALLING ASLEEP: Agar.
COUGH, TALKING, WHEN: Alum.; Phos.
COUGH, TICKLING: Bell.; Cham.; Phos.; Lyc.; Rhus t.
COUGH, VIOLENT: Phos.
COUGH, VIOLENT AFTER EVERY MEAL: China.
COUGH, WHOOPING: Cup.m.; Dros.
COUGH, WHOOPING WITH NAUSEA: Ipec.; Mag.p.
COUGH, WITH BURNING IN CHEST: Carb.v.
COUGH, WITH DIFFICULT RESPIRATION: Phos.
COUGH, WITH EXPECTORATION, OFFENSIVE: Bor.
COUGH, WITH FREQUENT SNEEZING: Alum.
COUGH, WITH PAIN IN HIP, BETTER COLD WATER: Caust.
COUGH, WITH PROFUSE YELLOW, STICKY MUCUS IN LONG
STRINGS: Kali b.
COUGH, WITH RAW CHEST: Caust.
COUGH, WITH SHORTNESS OF BREATH: Acon.; Alum.
COUGH, WITH SORE CHEST: Caust.
COUGH, WITH STITCHES IN CHEST: Merc.s.
COUGH, WITH STITCHING PAIN: Kali c.
COUGH, WITH VOMITING: Alum.
COUGH, WITH VOMITING OF FOOD: Ferr.m.
COUGH, WORSE AFTER DRINKING: Bry.; Spong.
COUGH, WORSE AFTER EATING: Bry.; Spong.
COUGH, WORSE NIGHT: Cimic.; Dros.
COUGH, WORSE SPEAKING: Cimic.
COUGH, WORSE WARM ROOM: Bry.; Ant.c.
COUGH, WORSE WARMTH OF BED: Caust.
COUGHING AND GAPING CONSECUTIVELY: Ant.t.
COUGHING MUST HOLD CHEST WHEN: Nat.s.

INSPIRATION DIFFICULT: Phos.ac.

RESPIRATION ANXIOUS: Phos.
RESPIRATION DIFFICULT: Phos.

RESPIRATION DIFFICULT FEELING OF PLUG IN
LARYNX: Spong.
RESPIRATION LABOURED: Phos.
RESPIRATION PAINFUL: Led.
RESPIRATION SIGHING: Op.
RESPIRATION WORSE SINGING: Spong.
RESPIRATION WORSE SWALLOWING: Spong.
RESPIRATION WORSE TALKING: Spong.

HEART

ACTION RAPID: **Cact.**
ACTION VIOLENT: **Cact.**
ANGINA PECTORIS: **Aur.; Mag.p.**
ANXIETY AROUND: **Phos.**

BLEEDS SUDDENLY INTO BLOOD VESSELS: **Ferr.m.**
BLOOD PRESSURE HIGH: **Aur.**

ENDOCARDITIS: **Cact.**

FLUTTERING: **Cact.**

INTERMITTENT HEARTBEAT: **Nat.m.**
IRREGULARITY OF HEART ACTION: **Cact.**

PALPITATION: **Cact.**
PALPITATION AND ANGUISH GOING UPSTAIRS: **Nit.a.**
PALPITATION AS FROM OBSTRUCTION: **Amb.g.**
PALPITATION IRREGULAR: **Agar.**
PALPITATION WITH ANXIETY: **Acon.**
PALPITATION WITH TINGLING IN FINGERS: **Acon.**
PALPITATION VIOLENT: **Glon.; Phos.**
PALPITATION VIOLENT CAN ONLY LIE ON RIGHT
SIDE: **Spig.**
PALPITATION VIOLENT CAN ONLY LIE WITH HEAD
HIGH: **Spig.**
PANTING: **Nit.a.**
PULSE BOUNDING: **Acon.**
PULSE FEEBLE: **Acon.**
PULSE FULL: **Acon.**
PULSE FULL BUT SOFT AND YIELDING: **Ferr.m.**
PULSE IRREGULAR: **Aur.**
PULSE RAPID: **Aur.**
PULSE RAPID IN MORNING: **Sul.**
PULSE SLOW: **Gels.**
PULSE SMALL AND WEAK: **Ferr.m.**
PULSE TENSE: **Acon.**
PULSE WEAK: **Gels.**

SENSATION AS IF HEART STOPPED BEATING: **Aur.**

SURGING OF HEART TO CHEST: Spong.

TROUBLES SOMETIMES CAUSED BY INFLAMMATORY
RHEUMATISM: Cact.

WEAK: Amm.c.

BACK

ACHE, WORSE MORNING BEFORE RISING AND AT NIGHT IN
BED: **Staph.**
ACHING, DULL: **Zinc.**
ACHING, LOW DOWN: **Nux v.**
ACHING, WITH NAUSEA: **Ipec.**

BEND, CANNOT: **Ruta.**

CONTRACTION OF: **Cimic.**

HEAVINESS IN: **Rhus t.**

PAIN IN: **Agar.**
PAIN IN SACRO-LUMBAR REGION: **Ant.t.**
PAIN IN SMALL OF: **Dulc.**
PAIN IN SMALL OF PARALYTIC: **Cocc.**
PAIN IN SPINE AS IF BEATEN: **Ruta.**
PAIN NEURALGIC: **Nit.a.**
PAIN SHARP GOING UP SPINE TO BACK OF HEAD: **Petr.**
PAIN STITCHING: **Bry.**
PAIN SUDDEN WHEN STOOPING: **Sep.**
PRESSURE IN: **Rhus t.**

SACRUM, PRESSURE OVER: **Hyper.**
SCIATICA: **Amm.m.**
SENSATION OF HEAVY WEIGHT IN COCCYX: **Ant.t.**
SPINE, CONCUSSION OF: **Hyper.**
STIFFNESS: **Bry.; Cimic.**
STIFFNESS IN SMALL OF: **Rhus t.**
STOOP-SHOULDERED: **Sul.**

EXTREMITIES

ACHING: Rhus t.
ACHING SORENESS: Bapt.
ARMS, CONTRACTION OF: Colo.
ARMS, MUSCLES, SORENESS: Cimic.
ARMS, MUSCLES, TEARING IN: Calc.c.
ARMS, MUSCLES, UNSTEADINESS OF FOREARM AND
HAND: Caust.
ARMS, NEURALGIA EXTENDING TO BOTH: Spig.
ARMS, PAIN, PRICKING IN: Apis
ARMS, SENSATION AS IF TOO SHORT: Amm.m.
ARMS, WRISTDROP: Plumb.

BONES, BROKEN, REFUSE TO KNIT: Calc.p.
BONES, BRUISING OF: Ruta.
BONES, FEELING AS IF SCRAPED WITH KNIFE: Phos.ac.
BONES, INFLAMMATION OF: Phos.ac.
BONES, MECHANICAL INJURIES OF: Ruta.
BONES, OF FEET PAINFUL AS IF BRUISED: Ruta.
BONES, OF HAND (BACK OF) PAINFUL: Ruta.
BONES, OF WRIST PAINFUL: Ruta.
BRUISED FEELING: Bapt.; Phos.ac.

CHILBLAINS: Agar.
CHOREA: Mag.p.
COLD: Arn.
COLD FROM KNEES DOWN: Carb.v.
CONVULSIONS: Nux v.; Stram.
CRURAL (THIGH) NEURALGIA: Staph

DEBILITY: Nit.a.

EVERYTHING ON WHICH HE LIES FEELS HARD FROM
BRUISING: Arn.

FEET COLD: Acon.; Apis.; Calc.c.
FEET COLD ICY: Dulc.
FEET COLD ICY IN BED: Sil.
FEET COLD ICY EVENING: Sil.
FEET CONSTANT MOTION IN: Zinc.
FEET CRAMPS IN: Cup.m.

FEET CRAWLING IN: **Hyper.**
FEET DAMP, FEEL: **Calc.c.**
FEET HEELS ACHING: **Phyt.**
FEET HEELS GOUT IN, WORSE TOUCH: **Colch.**
FEET HEELS NUMBNESS: **Alum.**
FEET HEELS PAIN AS IF ULCERATED: **Amm.c.**
FEET ITCHING OF, AS IF FROZEN: **Agar.**
FEET NUMBNESS: **Acon.; Apis.**
FEET OEDEMA IN: **Cact.**
FEET PERSPIRATION, OFTEN: **Sil.**
FEET SOLES OF, BURNING: **Sul.**
FEET SOLES OF, RAW: **Calc.c.**
FEET SOLES OF, SENSITIVE: **Kali c.**
FEET SWELLING OF: **Apis.**
FEET TINGLING: **Acon.**
FEET TOE, BIG, RIGHT, PAIN AT NIGHT: **Plumb.**
FEET, TOES BURN: **Apis.**
FEET, TOES INFLAMMATION OF BIG TOE, WORSE
TOUCH: **Colch.**
FEET, TOES ITCHING OF, AS IF FROZEN: **Agar.**
FEET, TOES PAINS IN, SHOOTING: **Amm.m.**
FEET, TOES PAINS IN, TEARING: **Amm.m.**
FEET, TREMBLING: **Apis.**
FEET, TWITCHING: **Stram.**
FINGER JOINTS, SWELLING OF: **Berb.**
FINGER NAILS BLACK: **Graph.**
FINGER NAILS BRITTLE: **Alum.**
FINGER NAILS OUT OF SHAPE: **Graph.**
FINGER NAILS ROUGH: **Graph.**
FINGER NAILS THICK: **Graph.**
FINGER NAILS UNDER, NEURALGIA: **Berb.**
FINGER TIPS COLD, ICY: **Chel.**
FINGER TIPS CRACKED: **Petr.**
FINGER TIPS FISSURED: **Petr.**
FINGER TIPS PAINS SHOOTING: **Amm.m.**
FINGER TIPS PAINS TEARING: **Amm.m.**
FINGER TIPS ROUGH: **Petr.**
FINGERS, NUMBNESS OF: **Amb.g.**
FINGERS, PAIN IN: **Ant.c.**

HANDS, CHILBLAINS ON: **Petr.**
HANDS, CRAMPS IN: **Amb.g.**
HANDS, CRAWLING IN: **Hyper.**

HANDS, HOT: Acon.; Agar.; Sul.

HANDS, ITCHING: Agar.

HANDS, NUMBNESS OF: Acon.; Apis.

HANDS, OEDEMA OF: Cact.

HANDS, RED: Agar.

HANDS, SWEATING: Sul.

HANDS, SWELLING OF: Agar.; Apis.

HANDS, TREMBLING: Agar.; Apis.; Merc.s.

HANDS, TWITCHING: Stram.

HEAVINESS OF: Nit.a.

HIPS, PAIN AS IF BRUISED: Ruta

HIPS, PAIN BURNING: Rhus t.

HIPS, PAIN CRAMP-LIKE: Colo.

HIPS, PAIN DARTING: Rhus t.

HIPS, PAIN EXCRUCIATING IN RIGHT JOINT: Nat.s.

HIPS, PAIN FROM HIP TO KNEE: Kali c.

HIPS, PAIN PRESSING: Rhus t.

HIPS, PAIN SHOOTING: Rhus t.

JERKING: Plumb.; Thuj.

JOINTS CRACK: Thuj.

JOINTS HOT: Bry.

JOINTS PAIN IN: Dros.

JOINTS PAINFUL AS IF BRUISED: Ruta.

JOINTS RED: Bry.

JOINTS SWOLLEN: Bry.

KNEELING CAUSES FAINTNESS: Sep.

KNEELING CAUSES PROSTRATION: Sep.

KNEES CRACK ON MOTION: Cocc.

KNEES PAIN IN: Kali c.

KNEES STIFFNESS OF: Rhus t.

LEGS, ANKLES, WEAKNESS: Nat.s.

LEGS, BEND GOING UP STAIRS: Ruta.

LEGS, CALVES, CRAMP IN: Cup.m.; Ver.a.

LEGS, CALVES RIGIDITY OF: Arg.n.

LEGS, EXHAUSTION ON WALKING: Phos.ac.

LEGS, PAIN, PRICKING: Apis.

LEGS, PAIN, TEARING IN BONES OF: Nit.a.

LEGS, RESTLESS: Ruta.

LEGS, RESTLESS AT NIGHT: Caust.

LEGS, VARICOSE VEINS IN: Zinc.

MUSCLES FEEL AS IF BEATEN: **Thuj.**

NEURITIS WITH BURNING: **Hyper.**
NEURITIS WITH TINGLING: **Hyper.**
NUMBNESS OF: **Plumb.**

OPERATIONS, SURGICAL, AFTER: **Staph.**

PAIN IN: **Cocc.**
PAINS BURNING: **Apis.**
PAINS DRIVING PATIENT OUT OF BED: **Thuj.**
PAINS GROWING: **Phos.ac.**
PAINS NEURALGIC: **Plumb.**
PAINS RHEUMATIC, LIKE ELECTRIC SHOCKS, SHIFTING
RAPIDLY: **Phyt.**
PAINS STITCHING, WORSE MOVEMENT: **Bry.**
PAINS TEARING, WORSE MOVEMENT: **Bry.**
PAINS VIOLENT: **Plumb.**
PAINS WITH COLD, NUMB FEELING: **Calc.p.**
PAINS WORSE MOVING IN BED: **Nat.c.**
PAINS WORSE SLIGHTEST TOUCH: **China.**
PARALYSIS OF SINGLE MUSCLES: **Plumb.**
PERIOSTITIS: **Ruta.**
PROSTRATION: **Bapt.**

RESTLESS: **Rhus t.**
RESTLESS CONSTANT: **Stram.**
RHEUMATIC TEARING IN LIMBS, BETTER WARMTH: **Caust.**
RHEUMATISM: **Aur.; Calc.p.**
RHEUMATISM ALTERNATING WITH CATARRH: **Kali b.**
RHEUMATISM ALTERNATING WITH STOMACH
TROUBLES: **Kali b.**
RHEUMATISM BEGINS IN FEET AND TRAVELS
UPWARDS: **Led.**
RHEUMATISM DRIVES PATIENT OUT OF BED: **Thuj.**
RHEUMATISM WANDERING: **Kali b.**

SCIATICA, PAINS RUN DOWN OUTER SIDE OF LIMBS: **Phyt.**
SCIATICA, WORSE ON RIGHT SIDE: **Lyc.**
SHOULDERS, COLDNESS BETWEEN, WITH CHEST
INFECTION: **Amm.m.**
SHOULDERS, COLDNESS IN BETWEEN: **Amm.m.**
SHOULDERS, PAIN AS IF BRUISED: **Cocc.**

SHOULDERS, PAIN BETWEEN BURNING: Lyc.; Phos.
SHOULDERS, PAIN IN JOINTS OF: Led.
SLEEP, GO TO: Carb.v.
SORE: Bapt.
SORENESS, WORSE TOUCH: Bry.
SPASMS BEGIN IN FINGERS AND TOES AND
SPREAD: Cup.m.
SPASMS TWITCHING: Nux v.; Zinc.
SPRAINS: Ruta.
STIFFNESS ALL OVER: Thuj.
STIFFNESS ON FIRST MOVING: Rhus t.
STIFFNESS WITH COLD, NUMB FEELING: Calc.p.
SWEATING ON SLIGHTEST MOTION: Agar.
SWEATING WHEN WALKING: Agar.

TENDONS CONTRACTED: Caust.
TENSION: Rhus t.
TREMBLING: Cocc.; Gels.; Nit.a.; Plumb.; Stram.; Zinc.

WEAKNESS, EXCESSIVE: Gels.
WEAKNESS, OF ALL: Merc.s.; Phos.; Rhus t.; Sil.; Zinc.
WOUNDS, CLEAN CUT AS AFTER SURGERY: Staph.

FEVER

ACTIVITY DURING: **Hyos.**
ATTACKS OF HEAT WITH ANXIETY: **Spong.**

CHILL AT 2 p.m.: **Calc.c.**
CHILL AT 4 p.m.: **Ferr.m.**
CHILL RUNS UP AND DOWN BACK, DURING: **Mag.p.**
CHILLINESS, EVENING: **Amm.m.**
CHILLINESS, PERSPIRATION AND HEAT OFF SKIN: **Cocc.**
COLDNESS: **Calen.**
COLDNESS EXTREME: **Ver.a.**

FLUSHES OF HEAT: **Sul.; Thuj.**

HEAD BURNING BUT REST OF BODY COLD: **Acon.**
HEAT, NAUSEA, VOMITING: **Ipec.**
HIGH FEVER: **Phyt.**

LOWER LEGS POWERLESS: **Rhus t.**

MALARIAL CONDITIONS: **Bapt.**

PERSPIRATION OFFENSIVE: **Merc.s.**
PERSPIRATION PROFUSE: **Merc.s.**
PULSE FULL AND SLOW: **Op.**

RESTLESSNESS: **Acon.; Hyos.; Rhus t.**
RESTLESSNESS GREAT: **Hyos.**

SENSITIVITY TO OPEN AIR, GREAT: **Calen.**
SEPTIC CONDITION OF BLOOD: **Bapt.**
SEPTIC FEVERS: **Bapt.**
SHAKES, BADLY, WANTS TO BE HELD: **Gels.**
SHIVERING: **Agar.; Mag.p.**
SHIVERING AND CHILLINESS ON SLIGHTEST MOVEMENT
OR EXPOSURE TO COLD AIR: **Nux v.**
STEAMING HEAT: **Acon.**
SWEATS AT NIGHT, ESPECIALLY HEAD, NECK AND
CHEST: **Calc.c.**
SWEATS ON HEAD IN CHILDREN: **Calc.c.**

THIRST: **Acon.**

UNCOVERING: **Hyos.**

WAVES OF COLD: **Acon.**
WAVES OF HEAT: **Acon.**
WEAKNESS: **Rhus t.**

SKIN

ABSCESS: **Led.**
AFFECTIONS FROM SUPPRESSED SKIN TROUBLES: **Cup.m.**
ANTS, FEELING OF, RUNNING ABOUT: **Phos.ac.**

BLEEDING: **Petr.**
BLUE: **Carb.v.; Cup.m.; Ver.a.**
BOILS, PAINFUL: **Arn.**
BOILS, SMALL: **Arn.**
BOILS, SORE: **Arn.**
BURNING: **Agar.; Bell.; Berb.; Rhus t.; Stram.; Sul.**
BURNS FOLLOWED BY UNDUE INFLAMMATION: **Canth.**
BURNS SCALD WITH RAWNESS: **Canth.**
BURNS SCALD WITH SMARTING: **Canth.**

CLAMMY: **Ver.a.**
COLD: **Carb.v.; China.; Ver.a.**
CRACKED: **Petr.**

DISCHARGE PROFUSE: **Thuj.**
DRY: **Colo.; Petr.; Sil.; Stram.**

ECZEMA: **Petr.; Rhus t.**
ECZEMA, EXCORIATING: **Rhus t.**
ECZEMA, OF ANUS: **Berb.**
ECZEMA, OF HANDS: **Berb.**
ECZEMA, OFFENSIVE: **Rhus t.**
ECZEMA, OOZING: **Rhus t.**
ECZEMA, RAW: **Rhus t.**
ECZEMA, WITH THICK CRUSTS: **Rhus t.**
ERUPTIONS, AFFECTS OF SUPPRESSED: **Strasm.**
ERUPTIONS, DRY ON MARGINS OF HAIR: **Nat.m.**
ERUPTIONS, HELPS TO BRING ON: **Gels.**
ERUPTIONS, ONLY ON COVERED PARTS: **Thuj.**
ERUPTIONS, OOZE STICKY SUBSTANCE: **Graph.**
ERUPTIONS, PUSTULAR: **Ant.t.**
ERUPTIONS, WITH BURNING: **Canth.**
ERUPTIONS, WITH ITCHING: **Canth.**
ERUPTIVE DISEASE, SEQUELAE WHEN ERUPTIONS FAIL TO
DEVELOP: **Apis.**
ERYSIPELAS: **Rhus t.; Ruta.**

EXCRESCENCES, CAULIFLOWER, SMELLING LIKE OLD
CHEESE OR HERRING BRINE: Thuj.

GREASY: Nat.m.

HEAT, FLUSHES OF: Sep.
HOT: Bell.; Colo.; Op.; Rhus t.; Stram.

INFLAMMATION OF: Apis.; China.
ITCHING: Agar.; Sul.
ITCHING INTENSE: Anac.; Berb.
ITCHING OF BODY AND HANDS: Phos.ac.
ITCHING OF PUPENDUM: Amb.g.
ITCHING WHEN GETTING WARM IN BED: Alum.

LEATHERY: Petr.

MARBLED: Cup.m.

NUMB: Calc.p.

OEDEMATOUS: Apis.

PAINS, BURNING: Rhus t.
PAINS, ITCHING: Rhus t.
PAINS, TINGLING: Rhus t.
PALE: Apis.; Bell.
PIGMENTATION, CIRCUMSCRIBED: Berb.

RASH, BURNING: Rhus t.
RASH, ITCHING: Rhus t.
RASH, RED: Rhus t.
RASH, SCRATCHING, NOT BETTER BY: Rhus t.
RASH, VESICULAR: Rhus t.
RED: Agar.; Apis.; Bell.
ROUGH: Petr.

SCALY: Sul.
SCARLET: Stram.
SENSATION OF BRUISING: Carb.v.
SENSATION OF CRAWLING: Carb.v.
SENSITIVE, BETTER HARD PRESSURE: China.
SENSITIVE, TO TOUCH: Apis.

SMARTING: Berb.
SORE: Apis.
SWEAT, SOUR SMELLING: Bry.
SWEATING: Sep.
SWEATING MORNING, EVERY: Phos.
SWEATING NERVOUS: Arg.n.
SWEATING NIGHT: Nit.a.; Sep.
SWEATING NIGHT TOWARDS MORNING: Sil.
SWEATING NIGHT WORSE: Bry.
SWEATING ON EXERTION, SLIGHT: Phos.
SWEATING OVER BODY EXCEPT LOWER LIMBS: Op.
SWEATING PROFUSE: Arg.n.; Bry.; China.; Phos.
SWEATING PROFUSE FROM LEAST EXERTION: Sep.
SWEATING RELIEF, BRINGS: Bry.
SWEATING SUDDEN: Arg.n.
SWELLING: Agar.
SWELLING ANYWHERE: Apis.

ULCERS, LARGE, BLEEDING: Merc.s.
ULCERS, PUTRID: Hep.s.
ULCERS, SENSITIVE, VERY: Hep.s.
UNHEALTHY: Graph.; Hep.s.; Sil.; Sul.
URTICARIA: Rhus t.
URTICARIA CHRONIC: Hep.s.
URTICARIA RECURRING: Hep.s.

WARTS: Thuj.
WAXY: Apis.
WOUNDS, PUNCTURE: Led.

YELLOW: Chel.

SLEEP

CATNAPS: **Sul.**

DELIRIUM WITH MUTTERING: **Agar.**
DELIRIUM WITH SHOUTING: **Agar.**
DELIRIUM WITH SINGING: **Agar.**
DROWSINESS: **Ant.t.; Apis.**
DROWSINESS DURING DAY: **Acon.**
DROWSINESS IN OLD PEOPLE: **Ant.c.**

INSOMNIA, NERVOUS: **Arg.n.**

RESTLESS: **Sil.**

SLEEP, DISTURBED AT NIGHT: **Acon.**
SLEEP, SCREAMS IN: **Apis.**
SLEEP, STARTS DURING: **Bell.**
SLEEP, STARTS SUDDENLY: **Apis.**
SLEEP, STARTS WHEN CLOSING EYES: **Bell.**
SLEEP, STARTS WHEN FEELING OF FALLING, TWITCHES,
WAKENS: **Agar.**
SLEEPINESS, CONSTANT EVEN IN DAY: **Phos.ac.**
SLEEPINESS, DURING DAY: **Amm.c.**
SLEEPLESS FROM WORRY: **Amb.g.**
SLUMBER, AROUSED BY SOME DISAGREEABLE
IDEAS: **Calc.c.**

WAKE UP, CAN HARDLY, IN MORNING: **Phos.ac.**
WAKES, FEELING FRIGHTENED AS IF
SUFFOCATING: **Spong.**
WAKES, SUDDENLY AFTER MIDNIGHT WITH PAIN AND
SUFFOCATION: **Spong.**
WAKES, TERRIFIED, SCREAMS: **Stram.**

MODALITIES

WORSE FROM or AGGRAVATED BY

ABDOMINAL SYMPTOMS, WORSE AFTERNOON: Amm.m.

ACIDS: Ant.c.

AIR, COLD: Calc.c.; Nux v.

AIR, COOL: Hep.s.

AIR, HOT: Lyc.

AIR, OPEN: Agar.; Carb.v.

ALCOHOLIC STIMULANTS: Sul.

ALONE, WHEN: Stram.

ALTERNATE DAYS: Lac.c.

ANGER: Cham.; Colo.; Staph.

ANYTHING UNUSUAL: Amb.g.

APPLICATIONS, COLD: Ars.

APPLICATIONS, HOT: Anac.

APPLICATIONS, OF HOT WATER: Anac.

APPLICATIONS, WARM: Lyc.

APPLICATIONS, WET: Amm.c.

APPROACH: Canth.

ASCENDING: Spong.

BATH, WARM: Lach.

BATHING: Calc.c.

BED, HOT: Lyc.

BED, WARM: Merc.s.; Sul.; Thuj.

BEER: Kali b.

BREAKFAST, AFTER: Thuj.

COFFEE: Carb.v.; Ign.; Kali c.; Thuj.

COITION, AFTER: Agar.; Kali c.

CONSOLATION: Nat.m.

CONSTRICTION: Lach.

CONTACT: Cup.m.

COOKING, SMELL OF: Colch.

DAY, EVERY OTHER: China.

DINNER, AFTER: Zinc.

DRAUGHTS: Bell.; Cham.; China.; Nat.c.; Sil.

DRINKING: Dros.

DRINKING COLD WATER: Canth.

DRINKING ICE COLD WATER WHEN HOT: Colo.

DRINKS, COLD: Ars.
DRINKS, HOT: Lach.
DRINKS, WARM: Phos.

EATING, AFTER: Agar.; Arg.n.; Cocc.; Kali p.; Nux v.; Puls
EATING, RAW FRUIT: Colo.
EMOTIONS: Arg.n.; Cocc.; Gels.
EXCITEMENT: Gels.; Kali p.
EXERTION: Anac.; Calc.c.; Kali p.; Phos.
EXERTION MENTAL: Calc.c.; Kali p.; Phos.
EXPOSURE, LEAST: Hyper.
EXPOSURE, TO GAS OR OPEN FIRE: Glon.
EXPOSURE TO SUN'S RAYS: Glon.
EYES, CLOSING: Lach.
EYES, MOVING: Spig.

FATS: Carb.v.
FLUIDS, LOSS OF: China.; Phos.ac.; Staph.
FOOD, COLD: Ars.
FOOD, FAT: Puls
FOOD, RICH: Puls.
FOOD, WARM: Phos.

GRIEF: Staph.

HAIR, CUT: Glon.
HEAT: Ant.c.; Bry.; Op.
HEATING, OVER: Ferr.m.

INDIGNATION: Colo.
INDOORS: Bapt.

JAR: Bell.; Cocc.; Glon.

LAUGHING: Dros.
LIGHT, BRIGHT: Thuj.
LIMBS, LETTING HANG DOWN: Calc.c.
LOOKING AT BRIGHT, SHINY OBJECTS: Stram.
LYING DOWN: Bell.; Dros.; Glon.; Hyos.; Ipec.; Nat.m.
LYING ON AFFECTED SIDE: Acon.; Hep.s.
LYING ON BACK: Rhus t.
LYING ON LEFT SIDE: Arg.n.; Cact.; Glon.; Kali c.; Lach.; Phos.;
Sil.

LYING ON PAINFUL SIDE: Amm.m.; Bar.c.; Kali c.; Phos.; Ruta.
LYING ON RIGHT SIDE: Chel.; Lyc.; Mag.p.; Merc.s.; Phyt.;
Rhus t.

MEALS, AFTER: Ign.
MENSES: Cocc.; Zinc.
MENSES BEFORE: Cham.; Cup.m.; Sep.
MENSES DURING: Arg.n.; Cham.; Hyos.; Sil.
MENTAL EXERTION: Anac.; Colch.; Nat.c.
MENTAL WORK: Nux v.
MENTAL STATES: Petr.
MILK: Carb.v.
MOON, FULL: Calc.c.; Sil.
MOON, NEW: Sil.
MORTIFICATION: Staph.
MOTION: Arn.; Berb.; Bry.; Chel.; Colch.; Phyt.; Plumb.
MOVEMENT, SLIGHTEST: Bry.
MUSIC: Amb.g.; Nat.c.

NARCOTICS: Thuj.
NEWS, BAD: Gels.
NOISE: Bell.; Cocc.; Spig.

PAIN, BY THINKING OF: Calc.p.
PERIODICALLY: Ipec.
POTATOES: Alum.
PRESSURE: Hep.s.; Lach.; Sil.
PRESSURE OF CLOTHES: Calc.c.

RADIATED HEAT: Ant.c.
REST, AT: Sul.
REST, DURING: Rhus t.; Ruta.
RIDING: Cocc.
ROOM, IN CLOSED: Hyper.
ROOM, IN COLD: Phyt.
ROOM, IN DARK: Stram.
ROOM, IN WARM: Acon.; Alum.; All.c.; Amb.g.; Lyc.; Puls.

SEA SHORE: Nat.m.
SEXUAL EXCESSES: Staph.
SIDE, LEFT: Arg.n.; Glon.; Lach.
SITTING: Nat.c.
SITTING STILL: Ferr.m.; Sep.

SLEEP, AFTER: Lac.c.; Lach.; Op.; Stram.
SLEEP, DURING: Op.
SLEEP, DURING WHEN AILMENTS BEGIN: Lach.
SLEEP, LOSS OF: Cocc.; Colch.
SMOKING: Cocc.; Ign.
SOUP: Kali c.
SPINE, PRESSURE ON DORSAL: Agar.
STANDING: Berb.; Sul.
STIMULANTS: Acon.; Nux v.
STOMACH EMPTY: Anac.
STOOPING: Glon.; Ruta.
STRANGERS, PRESENCE OF: Amb.g.
SUNDOWN TO SUNRISE: Colch.
SYMPTOMS FROM IMPEDED CIRCULATION: Phos.ac.
SWEAT, SUPPRESSED: Colo.
SWEATING: Ferr.m.; Merc.s.
SWEETS: Arg.n.
SWIMMING: Cocc.

TALKED TO: Phos.ac.
THINKING OF SYMPTOMS: Bar.c.
TIME 9 a.m.: Nux v.
TIME 10 a.m.: Gels.
TIME 10–11 a.m.: Nat.m.
TIME 11 a.m.: Cact.; Sul.
TIME 1–3 a.m.: Ars.
TIME 2–3 a.m.: Kali b.
TIME 3 a.m.: Kali c.
TIME 3–4 a.m.: Amm.c.
TIME 4–5 a.m.: Nat.s.
TIME 6 a.m. until noon: Glon.
TIME 4 p.m.: Colo.
TIME 4–8 p.m.: Lyc.
TIME 5–7 p.m.: Zinc.
TIME 11 p.m.: Cact.
TIME MIDNIGHT: Ferr.m.
TIME MIDNIGHT AFTER: Ars.; Calc.c.; Dros.
TIME MIDNIGHT BEFORE: Spong.
MORNING: Amb.g.; Alum.; Anac.; Bry.; Calc.c.; Ign.
MORNING EARLY: Chel.; Kali p.
MORNING LATE: Sep.
AFTERNOON: Agar.; Alum.; Bell.; Cocc.
EVENING: Amm.c.; Ant.c.

EVENING TOWARDS: Puls.
NIGHT: Amm.m.; Arg.n.; Ars.; Carb.v.; Dulc.; Hyos.; Lac.c.; Led.;
Mag.p.; Merc.s.; Nit.a.; Rhus t.; Thuj.; Ver.a.
NIGHT FIRST PART: Cham.
TOBACCO: Staph.
TOUCH: Bry.; Canth.; Chel.; Cocc.; Hyper.; Lac.c.; Mag.p.; Phos.;
Ruta.; Zinc.
TOUCH ON AFFECTED PARTS: Staph.
TOUCH SLIGHTEST: Arn.; Bell.; China.; Hep.s.
TOUCHED, BEING: Colch.

UPSTAIRS, GOING: Cact.
URINATING: Canth.

VEAL: Ipec.
VEHICLES, RIDING IN: Petr.

WAKING, ON: Alum.
WALKING: Cact.
WALKING OUT OF DOORS: Ruta.
WARMTH: Arg.n.; Bry.; Ign.; Puls.
WARMTH OF BED: Dros.
WASHING: Ant.c.; Bar.c.; Sep.; Sul.
WATER: Ant.c.
WEATHER, CHANGES FROM DAMP TO DRY: Sil.
WEATHER, CHANGES IN: Calc.p.; Chel.; Nat.c.
WEATHER, CLOUDY: Sep.
WEATHER, COLD: Agar.; Anac.; Aur.; Caust.; Hep.s.; Hyper.;
Kali c.; Kali p.; Mag.p.; Nit.a.
WEATHER, COLD AIR: Ars.; Calc.c.; Calc.p.; Carb.v.; Caust.;
Cimic.; Dulc.; Spig.; Thuj.; Ver.a.
WEATHER, COLD, DAMP: Arn.; Colo.
WEATHER, COLD, WET: Amm.c.
WEATHER, DAMP: Dulc.; Gels.; Hyper.; Merc.s.; Nat.s.; Petr.;
Phyt.; Rhus t.; Sep.; Spig.; Thuj.
WEATHER, DRY: Nux v.
WEATHER, DULL: Sep.
WEATHER, EXPOSURE TO COLD: Colch.
WEATHER, EXPOSURE TO DAMP: Colch.
WEATHER, FINE, CLEAR: Caust.
WEATHER, FOG: Bapt.; Hyper.
WEATHER, HEAT: Ant.c.; Bry.; Cham.; Kali b.; Lyc.; Nit.a.; Puls.
WEATHER, HEAT EXTREME: Colch.

WEATHER, HEAT HUMID: Bapt.
WEATHER, HEAT OF SUN: Ant.c.; Nat.m.
WEATHER, HEAT SUMMER: Nat.c.
WEATHER, RAINS, WHEN IT: Phyt.; Rhus t.; Spig.
WEATHER, SPRING: Lach.; Nat.s.
WEATHER, SUN: Nat.c.; Thuj.
WEATHER, SUNLIGHT: Acon.
WEATHER, TEMPERATURE, EXTREMES OF: Acon.
WEATHER, THUNDERSTORMS: Nat.c.; Petr.; Phos.; Sil.
WEATHER, THUNDERSTORMS BEFORE: Agar.; Sep.; Sil.
WEATHER, WARM: Bor.
WEATHER, WARM, WET: Carb.v.; Nat.s.
WEATHER, WARMTH AT NIGHT: Graph.
WEATHER, WET: Calc.c.; Ver.a.
WEATHER, WIND: Cham.
WEATHER, WIND COLD: Acon.; Colo.
WEATHER, WIND DRY: Acon.
WEATHER, WIND DRY COLD: Caust.; Hep.s.
WEATHER, WIND MOIST, WARM: Ipec.
WINTER: Petr.
WIND, IN: Spong.
WINE: Ant.c.; Arn.; Carb.v.; Glon.
WORRY: Kali p.

BETTER FROM or AMELIORATED BY
AIR, COLD: Puls.
AIR, COOL: Ant.t.; Bry.; Nat.s.; Thuj.
AIR, DRY: Spig.
AIR, OPEN: Acon.; All.c.; Alum.; Amm.m.; Ant.c.; Arg.n.; Cact.;
China.; Gels.; Lac.c.; Nat.m.; Phos.; Puls.
AIR, OPEN, SLOW MOTION IN: Amb.g.
ALTERNATE DAYS: Alum.
APPLICATIONS, COLD: Puls.
APPLICATIONS, COOL: Bry.
APPLICATIONS, HOT: Sil.
APPLICATIONS, WARM: Rhus t.

BACK, LYING ON: Calc.c.
BENDING DOUBLE: China.; Colo.; Mag.p.
BENDING FORWARD: Gels.
BENDING HEAD BACKWARDS: Hyper.
BORING IN EARS: Nat.c.

BORING IN NOSE: Nat.c.
BRANDY: Glon.
BREAKFAST, AFTER: Calc.c.; Staph.

CARRIED, BEING: Cham.
COLD: Arg.n.; Led.; Phos.
COLD BATHING: Nat.m.
COLD DRINKS: Amb.g.
COLD FOOD: Phos.
COLD FROM BEING UNCOVERED: Lyc.
COLD THINGS: Bry.; Op.
COLD WATER, FEET IN: Led.

COMPANY: Stram.
COOL ROOM: All.c.
COVERING: Nux v.

DARK, IN THE: Calc.c.; Graph.; Phos.
DAY, DURING: Kali c.
DESCENDING: Spong.
DISCHARGES: Zinc.
DRAWING UP AFFECTED LIMBS.:   Sul.
DRINKS, COLD: Puls.
DRINKS, WARM: Lyc.

EATING: Anac.; Ign.; Zinc.
ERUCTATIONS: Arg.n.; Carb.v.
ERUPTIONS, APPEARANCE OF: Zinc.
EXERCISE, BRISK: Sep.
EXERTION, PHYSICAL: Plumb.

FANNED, FROM BEING: Carb.v.
FOOD: Sep.
FOOD, COLD: Puls.
FOOD, WARM: Lyc.
FRICTION: Mag.p.

GARMENTS, LOOSENING OF: Calc.c.

HEADACHE BETTER BY PROFUSE URINATION: Gels.
HEAT: Kali b.

LIGHT, BRIGHT: Stram.

LIMBS, DRAWING UP: Calc.c.
LIMBS, STRETCHING: Rhus t.; Thuj.
LYING DOWN: Arn.; Lac.c.; Sil.
LYING MOTIONLESS: Bry.
LYING ON PAINFUL PARTS: Amb.g.
LYING ON PAINFUL SIDE: Bry.
LYING ON RIGHT SIDE: Nat.m.; Phos.; Sul.
LYING ON SIDE: Anac.
LYING QUIET: Cocc.

MASSAGED, BEING: Thuj.
MEAL, AFTER A: Hep.s.
MIDNIGHT, AFTER: Lyc.
MOTION: Gels.; Kali c.; Lyc.; Nat.c.; Rhus t.; Ruta.
MOVING ABOUT: Dulc.
MOVING ABOUT SLOWLY: Agar.

NAP, IF ALLOWED TO FINISH: Nux v.
NIGHT: Staph.
NOURISHMENT: Kali p.

PERSPIRATION, DURING: Cup.m.
POSITION, CHANGE OF: Ign.; Rhus t.
PRESSURE: Arg.n.; Arn.; Bry.; Chel.; Mag.p.
PRESSURE AGAINST BACK: Nat.m.
PRESSURE HARD: China.; Colo.; Plumb.; Sep.

QUIET: Spig.

REST, FROM: Anac.; Ant.c.; Calc.p.; Colch.; Kali p.; Lac.c.; Phyt.;
Staph.
RIDING IN VEHICLE: Cham.; Nit.a.
RISING, AFTER: Ferr.m.
RUBBING: Anac.; Calc.c.; Canth.; Plumb.; Rhus t.

SCRATCHING: Thuj.
SEMI-ERECT: Bell.
SLEEP, FROM: Acon.; Phos.; Sep.
SLEEP, SHORT, AFTER: Phos.ac.
STOOL, AFTER: Nux v.
STOOPING: Hyos.
SUMMER: Sil.
SUN, SETTING: Spig.

SWEATING, AFTER: Bry.; Thuj.
SWEATING, PROFUSE: Acon.

WALKING: Op.; Rhus t.; Ver.a.
WALKING AGAINST WIND: Sep.
WALKING IN OPEN AIR: Bar.c.
WALKING SLOWLY, BUT WEAKNESS FORCES HIM TO LIE
DOWN: Ferr.m.
WARMLY WRAPPED UP: Colch.; Sul.
WARMTH: Cimic.; Colch.; Colo.; Dulc.; Hep.s.; Kali p.; Lac.c.;
Mag.p.; Phos.ac.; Phyt.; Ruta.; Staph.; Stram.; Ver.a.
WARMTH EXCEPT HEAD: Ars.
WARMTH OF BED: Sep.
WASHING: Amm.c.
WASHING IN COLD WATER: Alum.; Phos.
WEATHER, COLD: Bor.; Carb.v.
WEATHER, DAMP: Alum.
WEATHER, DAMP MOIST: Ant.c.
WEATHER, DAMP WET: Caust.
WEATHER, DRY: Amm.c.; Calc.c.; Nat.s.; Petr.; Phyt.; Rhus t.;
Sul.
WEATHER, WARM: Calc.c.; China.; Rhus t.; Sul.
WEATHER, WARM MOIST: Kali c.
WEATHER, WARM MOIST HUMID: Cham.
WEATHER, WARM WET: Hep.s.
WEATHER, WET: Nux v.
WRAPPING UP: Graph.